*N*ursing *Theory*

UTILIZATION & APPLICATION

Nursing *Theory*
UTILIZATION & APPLICATION

Martha Raile Alligood, PhD, RN

Professor, College of Nursing, University of Tennessee,
Knoxville, Tennessee

Ann Marriner-Tomey, PhD, RN, FAAN

Professor and Dean, School of Nursing, Indiana State University,
Terre Haute, Indiana

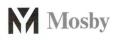 Mosby

St. Louis Baltimore Boston Carlsbad Chicago Naples New York Philadelphia Portland
London Madrid Mexico City Singapore Sydney Tokyo Toronto Wiesbaden

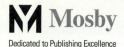

Mosby
Dedicated to Publishing Excellence

A Times Mirror Company

Publisher: Nancy L. Coon
Editor: Loren S. Wilson
Developmental Editor: Brian Dennison
Project Manager: Linda McKinley
Production Editor: Catherine Bricker
Editing and Production: Top Graphics
Designer: Jeanne Wolfgeher
Design Manager: Elizabeth Fett
Manufacturing Manager: Linda Ierardi

Printed in the United States of America
Composition by Top Graphics
Printing/binding by R. R. Donnelley & Sons Company

Mosby–Year Book, Inc.
11830 Westline Industrial Drive
St. Louis, Missouri 63146

Library of Congress Cataloging in Publication Data

Nursing theory : utilization and application / [edited by] Martha
  Raile Alligood, Ann Marriner-Tomey.
       p.   cm.
    Includes bibliographical references and index.
    ISBN 0-8151-0812-5 (pbk.)c
    1. Nursing models.   2. Nursing—Philosophy.   I. Alligood, Martha
Raile.   II. Marriner-Tomey, Ann, 1943-
    [DNLM: 1. Nursing Theory.   2. Models, Nursing.   WY 86 N9758 1997]
RT84.5.N94 1997
610.73—dc20
DNLM/DLC
for Library of Congress   96-19839
                                                                         CIP

96 97 98 99 00 / 9 8 7 6 5 4 3 2 1

Contributors

Martha Raile Alligood, PhD, RN
Professor, College of Nursing,
University of Tennessee,
Knoxville, Tennessee

Violeta A. Berbiglia, EdD, RN
Associate Professor,
Texas A&M University at Corpus Christi,
Corpus Christi, Texas

Kaye Bultemeier, PhD, RNCS
Family Nurse Practitioner,
Women's Health Associates,
Oak Ridge, Tennessee

Jacqueline Fawcett, PhD, FAAN
Professor, School of Nursing,
University of Pennsylvania,
Philadelphia, Pennsylvania

Maureen A. Frey, PhD, RN
Director of Nursing Research/
  Advanced Practice,
Children's Hospital of Michigan,
Detroit, Michigan

Bonnie Holaday, DNS, RN, FAAN
Professor and Chair, School of Nursing,
Wichita State University,
Wichita, Kansas

Diane Norris, MSN, RN
Project Nurse Manager,
Children's Hospital of Michigan,
Detroit, Michigan

Kenneth D. Phillips, PhD, RN
Assistant Professor, College of Nursing,
University of South Carolina,
Columbia, South Carolina

Karen Moore Schaefer, DNSc, RN
Associate Professor,
Allentown College of St. Francis de Sales,
Center Valley, Pennsylvania

Raphella Sohier, PhD, RN
Professor,
MGH Institute of Health Professions
  at Massachusetts General Hospital,
Boston, Massachusetts

To our mothers,
   Winifred Raile, RN
   and
   Arlene Clawson

and our husbands,
   Charlie K. Alligood
   and
   H. Keith Tomey

Preface

Nursing Theory: Utilization and Application was written to provide students and nurses with a text that demonstrates how theory guides nursing practice. The text builds on two premises: (1) the nature of knowledge needed for the practice of nursing is theoretical and (2) practice is central to nursing. On these foundations, the phase of utilization and application of theory is essential to the ongoing, knowledge-building process of a practice discipline such as nursing.

This text may be used to teach nurses and student nurses how nursing models and their theories guide the critical thinking process of professional nursing practice. It will be useful to those individuals teaching theory-based nursing practice in baccalaureate nursing programs, in-service education programs, and graduate-level nursing courses on the theoretical foundations of nursing and advanced practice clinical nursing.

Although *Nursing Theory: Utilization and Application* builds on the idea that nursing practice needs to move beyond theory analysis to theory utilization, the student using the text needs a basic understanding of nursing models and theories. Therefore a companion text such as *Nursing Theorists and Their Work* is suggested, which introduces the reader to nursing philosophies, models, and theories and clearly links them to nursing practice. For example, students can review a corresponding chapter in the companion book for a basic understanding of the model as background for the chapter on its use in practice in *Nursing Theory: Utilization and Application*.

ORGANIZATION

The content of the book is presented in three parts with the following features:

Part I puts the theme of the text, which is the use of theory to guide nursing practice, into a usable context. Chapter 1 provides a historical background for the century of professional development that has led to the present phase of the theory era. The quest for nursing knowledge is viewed as a driving force that has shaped the nursing profession. Chapter 2 reviews areas in which theory-based nursing practice has been reported in the nursing literature. Three tables are presented that illustrate the wide use of theory-based practice in various areas in which nursing is practiced. Chapter 3 presents models and theories as critical thinking structures from a structure of knowledge perspective. In addition, the major models and their theories are reviewed, clarifying the utility of middle-range theory for application in professional nursing practice, and guidelines are provided for the student's use in selecting a nursing model or theory for practice.

Part II is the heart of the text, with seven chapters (4 through 10) that demonstrate the utilization and application of models as critical thinking structures in clinical cases. The chapters are written by clinical experts who apply the models to the nursing care of a hypothetical patient named Debbie and another case selected from their practice. Each of these chapters features a table that aligns the content focus of a particular model with the critical thinking process associated with that model. Critical thinking exercises are presented in each chapter to assist students with utilization and application of a model and its theories in their own nursing practice.

Part III features Chapters 11 and 12, which emphasize the need for expansion of theory-based nursing practice. Chapter 11 mirrors Chapter 2 and identifies areas in which theory-based practice has not been reported and that can be expanded to include the use of the models and their theories. In addition, middle-range theories are proposed for these areas based on specific nursing situations, such as nursing actions, client population, and area of practice. Chapter 12 provides guidelines for transforming practice by changing perspectives.

Special features of the book include the following:
• Cases that illustrate application in nursing practice
• Use of the same case (Debbie) in Chapters 4 through 10
• Critical thinking with each model in the form of a table
• Critical thinking exercises at the end of each application chapter
• Glossary

• • •

We believe this is a useful text for undergraduate programs because of the emphasis on theory use. Because theory is presented as a guide for reasoning and decision making, the critical thinking process of professional practice becomes more clear. Major nursing models and their theories are applied to clinical cases to illustrate their utilization and application in the practice of nursing. Nursing faculty who want to emphasize nursing approaches to nursing practice in their teaching will find this text clear and direct.

For core theory courses in masters programs the text is useful in combination with a text such as the previously mentioned *Nursing Theorists and Their Work.* Nursing faculty who want to move their students beyond a survey of nursing model analyses to application of the models in practice will find that this text provides a basis for theory-based practice. Case examples that illustrate utilization and application of theory and practical ideas for the future expansion of theory-based nursing practice will help faculty make this transition.

ACKNOWLEDGMENTS

We would like to take this opportunity to thank the staff at Mosby for their work and support; the reviewers, Susan Rush Michael, RN, DNSc, CDE, Patricia H. Murphy, RN, EdD, CCRN, CRRN, and Carole Ann Pepa, RN, PhD, for their thoughtful suggestions; and the chapter contributors for their expert clinical and theoretical knowledge, with a special thank you to Dr. Kenneth D. Phillips for developing the case history of Debbie for this text and Dr. Jacqueline Fawcett who contributed a chapter and whose publications facilitated identifying the recent theory-based nursing practice literature.

Martha Raile Alligood
Ann Marriner-Tomey

Contents

PART I *Conceptualization,* 1

1 *The Nature of Knowledge Needed for Nursing Practice, 3*
MARTHA RAILE ALLIGOOD

2 *Models and Theories in Nursing Practice, 15*
MARTHA RAILE ALLIGOOD

3 *Models and Theories: Critical Thinking Structures, 31*
MARTHA RAILE ALLIGOOD

PART II *Application,* 47

4 *Johnson's Behavioral System Model in Nursing Practice, 49*
BONNIE HOLADAY

5 *King's Systems Framework and Theory in Nursing Practice, 71*
MAUREEN A. FREY
DIANE NORRIS

6 *Levine's Conservation Model in Nursing Practice, 89*
KAREN MOORE SCHAEFER

7 *Neuman's Systems Model in Nursing Practice, 109*
RAPHELLA SOHIER

8 *Orem's Self-Care Deficit Theory in Nursing Practice, 129*
VIOLETA A. BERBIGLIA

9 *Rogers' Science of Unitary Human Beings in Nursing Practice, 153*
KAYE BULTEMEIER

10 *Roy's Adaptation Model in Nursing Practice, 175*
KENNETH D. PHILLIPS

PART III   *Expansion,* 201

    11   *Areas for Further Development of Theory-Based Nursing Practice,* 203
        MARTHA RAILE ALLIGOOD

    12   *Conceptual Models of Nursing, Nursing Theories, and Nursing Practice: Focus on the Future,* 211
        JACQUELINE FAWCETT

    Glossary, 223

Nursing Theory
UTILIZATION & APPLICATION

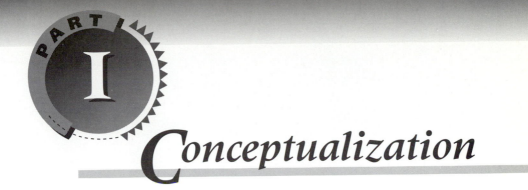

PART I

Conceptualization

Conceptualizations that provide the context for the premises of the text are:

- Nursing's century-long search for a substantive body of knowledge has led to a science of nursing that is of a theoretical nature.
- Practice is central to nursing.
- Theory utilization sheds new light on the theory-research-practice relationship.
- Nursing models are paradigms from which theories are derived to specify nursing approaches, actions, and outcomes.
- Model and theory utilization is visible in many areas of nursing practice.
- Nursing models and theories guide the reasoning process of critical thinking for professional nursing practice.

The Nature of Knowledge Needed for Nursing Practice

Martha Raile Alligood

"The systematic accumulation of knowledge is essential to progress in any profession . . . however, theory and practice must be constantly interactive. Theory without practice is empty and practice without theory is blind." (Cross, 1981)

This chapter highlights nursing's efforts toward the development of a body of knowledge to guide nursing practice in this century. Comprehension of the nursing model and nursing theory relationship clarifies the role of theory in relation to nursing practice. Theory informs the focus and content of practice as well as guides nursing action. Utilization of nursing models and their theories is presented as a means of organizing the reasoning process for critical thinking in professional nursing practice.

With the turn of the century, nursing began to move from vocation toward profession (Alligood, 1994a; Alligood, 1994b; Johnson, 1974; Kalish & Kalish, 1995; Meleis, 1991; Rogers, 1961). Guided by the words of Nightingale and the goal of professionalism, American nurses began to enter academia seeking higher education, first in individual courses and then in collegiate nursing programs. The background of this movement toward professionalism is important to consider in order to understand the different emphases the search for a body of knowledge has taken over the decades.

These different emphases have been viewed as eras in the history of nursing's march toward professionalism (Meleis, 1991). However, one criterion for the consideration of nursing as a profession has been a constant force in this development. That criterion specifies that nursing practice be guided by a body of specialized knowledge (Bixler & Bixler, 1959). Today our discussions are far beyond those of nursing becoming recognized as a profession, yet the criterion that calls for the utilization of a specialized body of knowledge to guide nursing practice continues to be evident. Clearly it has been the most pertinent criterion to the development of nursing as a profession.

A review of the efforts toward meeting the criterion lends clarity to the efforts of these eras and restores practice as nursing's central concern. Nursing's quest to answer the question of the nature of knowledge needed for the practice of nursing may be viewed as a driving force that has shaped our profession by guiding nurses and students of nursing in various directions that were often not clear nor completely understood at the time.

ERAS OF NURSING KNOWLEDGE

From the turn of the last century, the idea that nurses needed knowledge to guide and improve nursing practice is noted. Signs of a beginning national consciousness for nursing may be traced back to the first national gathering of nurses at the World's Fair in Chicago in 1893 and to the publication of the first edition of the *American Journal of Nursing (AJN),* the first national organ of communication for nurses, in October 1900 (Kalish & Kalish, 1995). From these initial national efforts of nurses, the goal to move nursing to the professional level began to emerge.

At this early time, the focus was on practice and teaching students to *do* nursing. These beginnings suggest, however, a move in the direction of recognizing the need for specialized knowledge to guide the practice of nursing. The journal *AJN* may be seen as an early symbol of nursing's movement toward becoming a profession and as evidence that nurses needed to interact with each other about nursing practice as well as about how to train nurses or teach nursing to others. With the boom of the industrial age, hospital training schools flourished in America and the curriculum era of the 1920s and 1930s soon followed (Kalish & Kalish, 1995).

Curriculum Era

In this era, efforts to answer the question of the nature of the knowledge needed for nursing practice are evident from the emphasis on content and movement toward the goal of standardization of curricula. The focus of this era is evident in state activities such as the 1933 survey of New York training schools regarding their curricula (Kalish & Kalish,

1995). It was this emphasis on what nurses needed to know in order to practice nursing that led to the expansion of curricula beyond medical knowledge to include social sciences and nursing procedures. The fact that these classes were often called "fundamentals," which means basic essentials, may reflect an early valuing of nursing content specific to nursing action in this era. Nursing's beginning embrace of science is also evident in the curricula of this early era.

It is interesting to note that nursing procedures were taught and practiced in a ward-type room called the "nursing arts" laboratory. When in later decades nursing curricula emphasized science and research, these rooms were referred to as "skills" laboratories. Reference to the art of nursing became unpopular and scarce in the nursing literature for a period of nursing's history. We are indebted to those scholars who maintained an emphasis on the art of nursing in this period as science gained popularity (Kalish & Kalish, 1995). The change in terminology may also be related to the beginning of baccalaureate nursing programs in this era because with the move of nursing into schools of higher learning, nursing was increasingly considered a science (Kalish & Kalish, 1995).

Once nursing began to be taught in colleges and universities, all of nursing was affected by that move into academe since nurses had to consider what that move meant with regard to them and the question of the nature of the knowledge needed for nursing and the body of knowledge needed to guide nursing practice. The move of nursing into higher education was a major shift for the nursing profession; the effects of this transition are still being felt today as nurses debate about multiple levels of entry into nursing practice.

Nursing leaders in this era were advocating that nursing needed to be taught in a different educational environment and at a different level of education. The move of nursing into schools of higher learning brought with it a significant change in the search for a substantive body of knowledge and led to the research era.

Research Era

In the 1940s and 1950s, research became the driving force. Nurses were on the move to conduct research and to begin developing that specialized body of knowledge. The task was so great, however, that it often became an end in itself. Learning to carry out research led to an emphasis on statistics and research methods, which were new areas of curriculum content that needed to be mastered. It was believed that research alone would generate the body of knowledge or science needed as a basis for nursing practice.

During this era there was an emphasis on scholarship and the need to disseminate research findings in scholarly publications. *Nursing Research,* the first nursing research journal, was established for this purpose in 1952. Two programs funded by the federal government were instituted in 1955 to prepare nurses as researchers and teachers of research: the United States Public Health Service predoctoral research fellowships and the Nurse Scientist Training Program (Schlotfeldt, 1992).

These research beginnings influenced nursing such that by the 1960s and 1970s, as more and more nurse educators were introduced to research, a new emphasis on graduate education in nursing was emerging, with nursing research included in curricula. The research and graduate education eras seem to overlap as has been noted by other reviewers (Meleis, 1991; Styles, 1982). The strong emphasis on nursing scholarship during both eras no doubt contributes to the blending and close interrelationship of the two eras (Fawcett, 1978).

Graduate Education Era

During the graduate education era of the 1960s and 1970s, curricula were proposed for masters-level preparation by regional groups and then standardized at national meetings of the National League for Nursing (NLN) such that by the end of the 1970s most accredited masters education programs in nursing included courses in nursing research, clinical specialty advanced practice, advanced physiology, and leadership. Many also included a course in nursing theory in a core curriculum organized with a nursing philosophy and conceptual framework.

Although there were only three nursing doctoral programs at the beginning of this era, the continuing post–World War II shortage of nurses, which had led to the federally funded programs in the 1950s, meant that nurses with doctorates from a wide range of related disciplines were being prepared for research and teaching roles in nursing. Therefore, although the American Nurses Association (ANA) had identified the need for nursing theory development in 1965, there was only general consensus as to what that meant because of the variety of discipline perspectives held by nurses with doctorates.

During this era, a series of three national conferences brought nurses together to exchange ideas and evaluate the results of their doctoral programs in other fields for nursing's needs. The papers and discussions from these conferences were published in *Nursing Research* in 1968 and 1969 and they were republished in Nicoll's first edition (1986) under the unit heading "Three Landmark Symposia" (p. 91). The conferences, which centered on nursing science and theory development, were designed to facilitate the discussion of the application of knowledge from the various disciplines to nursing. The Nurse Scientist program is noteworthy in this history because it dealt directly with the question of the nature of the body of nursing knowledge, that is, will nursing be other-discipline based or nursing based? Dealing with this question was a turning point for nursing with regard to graduate education and understanding of the nature of the body of knowledge needed for nursing practice.

Doctoral education began to flourish such that by the end of the 1970s there were 21 nursing doctoral programs and several more universities indicating the intent to develop programs. The driving force was no doubt the need to develop a specialized body of knowledge and the conclusion that it should be developed by nurses prepared in the discipline of nursing. Therefore it is not surprising that in this era a distinction was made between nursing knowledge and borrowed knowledge in the nursing literature (Johnson, 1968). This awareness grew out of the understanding that theory from other disciplines was not specific to nursing and its nursing knowledge needs (Johnson, 1968; Rogers, 1970).

During this era the theorists began publishing their nursing frameworks. The works by Johnson (1980), King (1971), Levine (1967), Neuman (1972), Orem (1971), Rogers (1970), and Roy (1970) were evidence of the new emphasis on nursing theory.

Research continued to develop during this era of graduate education; however, the knowledge generated was noted to lack form and direction. In fact, *Nursing Research* celebrated its 25th anniversary in 1977 (vol. 26, no. 3) with published reviews of the research progress. These reviews presented recommendations for development in five practice areas of nursing: medical-surgical, community, maternal-child, psychiatric, and gerontology. In general, the lack of conceptual or theoretical direction or connection in the research was identified as a weakness of the studies. It was also noted that the research focused on nurses or student nurses rather than on the patient.

From a comprehensive review of those first 25 years of published nursing research, Batey (1977) identified conceptualization as the greatest limitation of the projects. She emphasized the importance of the conceptual phase of research to provide a content basis as well as a connection with other studies to develop nursing science. It should be noted that reference to concepts and conceptualization was more common in this era and may now be considered a precursor to the theory era with the understanding of theory as a set of related concepts.

An indication of the shift of emphasis from research to theory at the national level began to be noted with the Nurse Educator conferences in Chicago (1977) and New York (1978). Although the first conference did not have a theory theme, Sr. Callista Roy's workshop on how to use her conceptual framework as a guide for nursing practice was so popular that the second conference was planned with a nursing theory theme and brought nursing theorists together on the same stage for the first time in history. That second conference underscored a growing awareness that the nature of the knowledge needed for nursing practice was theoretical knowledge.

Other factors in the shift toward theory at this time were the publication of Carper's patterns of knowing for nursing (1978) and Fawcett's article on the double-helix relationship between theory and research (1978) in the first edition of a new nursing journal, *Advances in Nursing Science*. Carper (1978) identified four types of nursing knowledge and clarified their contexts. Her work is significant in this history for distinguishing empirical knowledge from ethical, personal, and aesthetic. In the same issue, Fawcett (1978) clarified the relationship of theory and research in the development of science in her classic double-helix metaphor presentation. These events ushered in the theory era of the 1980s and 1990s.

Theory Era

The theory era began with a strong emphasis on development. Although the previous two decades had proponents of nursing theory and the nursing theorists had begun to publish their frameworks, it is noteworthy that they denied being theorists when they were introduced at the Nurse Educator theory conference in 1978. There was a strong sense among those attending the conference that they were theorists, and by the second day the audience responded to their denials with laughter.

In only one decade—from 1980 to 1990—nursing theory development stimulated phenomenal growth, which has been noted to be the cornerstone of the development of the discipline of nursing (Meleis, 1983). The theory era coupled with the research era led to an understanding of the scientific process for the production of a scientific product (Whall, 1989). This era stimulated the growth of nursing scholarship in a way never before experienced in nursing history (Schlotfeldt, 1992). Proliferation of nursing literature and new nursing journals, national and international nursing conferences, and the opening of new nursing doctoral programs are evidence of the growth of this era.

Also during this decade, Fawcett (1984, 1989) made a significant contribution to our understanding of the nature of nursing knowledge. She developed a metaparadigm explanation of the interconnectedness of the various nursing theoretical works and proposed a structure of nursing knowledge according to Kuhn's philosophy of science (1970), which began to clarify different levels of abstraction in nursing theoretical works. Her work is particularly significant to this history because the structure she proposed led to an understanding of middle-range or practice theory for the theory utilization phase of the theory era. Although Fawcett's work focuses on analysis and evaluation of nursing models and theories, her structure demonstrates the decreasing level of abstraction in the direction of nursing practice. Most important, the structure shows how nursing theory is connected to or is derived from the models of nursing. This interconnection of nursing knowledge is vital to the development of nursing science.

It is important to note that the emphasis on theory development was only a phase of the theory era, which focused on the process of knowledge development. Although necessary for our understanding, analysis and critique of the process or syntax and structure alone will not tell about the use of the model or theory in practice. Therefore there is a need to shift the emphasis from theory development to theory utilization because the real value of theory for nursing practice will be known only from using it in practice. Knowledge pertinent to further theory development and continued progress of nursing as a professional discipline will also be gained in this phase of the era (Whall, 1989).

This text recognizes the significance of the changing emphasis from theory *development* to theory *utilization*. From the perspective of theory utilization, the earlier eras begin to be seen in a different light. That is, we come to understand that curriculum and education were very important but they were not an end. Likewise, research, as important as it was to nursing's growth, was not an end nor would research alone produce science but required an interrelationship with theory to do so (Fawcett, 1978). Theory is not an end either, although it might have seemed so during the past decade considering the strong emphasis it received. Rather, theory and research together lead to science, which informs practice.

Education, research, and theory are all understood in this new alignment as tools of nursing practice. Only by clarifying the relationship of these important processes to nursing practice can nurses properly use them to advance the discipline. Theory utilization reestablishes practice as the central focus for the discipline of nursing. This text emphasizes nursing practice with a focus on knowledge utilization, clarifying theory and research as tools of practice (Alligood, 1994b; Allison, McLaughlin, & Walker, 1991; Field, 1987).

This position is in concert with the national agenda to move education from lower order learning with a recall focus to higher order learning with a reasoning focus. The Council of Baccalaureate and Higher Degree Programs (CBHDP) of the National League for Nursing (NLN) joined ranks with this initiative in the development of the latest set of criteria (1992) for accrediting member programs. The National Council for Excellence in Critical Thinking Instruction (Paul & Nosich, 1991) defines critical thinking as "the intellectually disciplined process of actively and skillfully conceptualizing, applying, analyzing, synthesizing or evaluating information gathered from, or generated by, observation, experience, reflection, reasoning, or communication, as a guide to belief and action" (p. 4). This text presents utilization of the nursing models and their theories as guides for the reasoning and decision-making process and information-processing skills for substantive critical thinking. Nursing theory becomes a critical thinking structure to specify the focus and guide the clinical decision-making process of professional nursing practice.

• • •

In summary, nursing's search for a specialized body of nursing knowledge has been evident most of this century. In the early era of the 1920s and 1930s, the emphasis was on curriculum and nursing education and nursing experienced a phenomenal expansion of nursing programs with an emphasis on nursing procedures and training for basic nursing. In the era of the 1940s and 1950s, nursing began the move into higher education, graduate programs were developed, and nursing research began to be conducted as nursing developed as a scientific discipline. In the 1960s and 1970s, the experiment of preparing nurse scientists in other disciplines ended and the direction for the development of the discipline was clarified, leading to an immediate expansion of nursing doctoral programs. The era of the 1980s and 1990s began with a theory development emphasis, which is now shifting to theory utilization.

This brief history suggests how the emphasis of each era of nursing history led to a limited vision or partial view of where the discipline was headed. The point must be made that each of these eras was necessary for the growth and development of nursing and that movement is necessary for the continued growth of nursing as a discipline.

CENTRALITY OF NURSING PRACTICE

The premise that practice is central to nursing is vital. This text is an answer to the question: "What is the nature of the knowledge that is needed for the practice of nursing?" This question has been a driving force for the nursing profession since its origin. Nursing history suggests that it was in dealing with this question that the eras of growth have occurred. Although nursing practice has continued throughout these eras, efforts have often been divided. The proper focus on nursing practice will facilitate nursing unity for continued professional development and pave the way for the recognition of professional nurses as key players in the healthcare delivery systems of the next century.

For nurses to make their contribution, it is essential they practice nursing in an organized manner. Nurses need to move beyond practice conventions to interventions using nursing models that are holistic and nursing based rather than focused on physiological and psychosocial concerns (Sparacino, 1991). This move requires an approach to care that is consciously defined (Wardle & Mandle, 1989). The analytical process and complex reasoning for nursing judgments do not come automatically as Wardle & Mandle (1989) found in their study of the frameworks nurses use in nursing practice. Rather, theory utilization requires knowledge and skill in practice. Furthermore, nursing needs to be practiced in a relationship with the patient rather than with the limited cross-sectional approach of the medical model (Alligood, 1994b).

Utilization of nursing theory, applied in nursing practice, provides a framework for a nursing approach and guides the critical thinking process of reasoning and decision making for nurses to practice in an organized manner. The nursing literature continues to echo the urgent need for theory to guide nursing practice (Algase & Whall, 1993). Mathwig (1975) said even before the theory era that the first phase of translating theory into practice is the decision to do so. Similarly, use of a model in practice has been described as a habit to be formed (Broncatello, 1980), the practice of a true believer (Oliver, 1991), and the practice of one who has been properly persuaded (Levine, 1995).

The delay in moving into theory utilization is best explained by nursing history. Change comes slow and is greatly influenced by the eras preceding it, but it does come. The application of theory in practice has been described as the acid test for theory since the mark of its usefulness is its ability to guide practice (Martin, Forchuk, Santopinto, & Butcher, 1992). That understanding has led authors to declare that it is essential that these models be tested and that testing be done in a variety of settings (Huckabay, 1991; Whall, 1989). The theory utilization phase of the theory era will usher in the next era of nursing history, which will be an era of theory testing through application in practice and will further contribute to professional nursing development (Fawcett, 1995).

References

Algase, D. L., & Whall, A. F. (1993). Rosemary Ellis' views on the substantive structure of nursing. *IMAGE: Journal of Nursing Scholarship, 25*(1), 69-72.

Alligood, M. R. (1994a). Evolution of nursing theory development. In A Marriner-Tomey, (Ed.), *Nursing theorists and their work* (3rd ed., pp. 58-69). St. Louis: Mosby.

Alligood, M. R. (1994b). Toward a unitary view of nursing practice. In M. Madrid & E. A. M. Barrett (Eds.), *Rogers' scientific art of nursing practice* (pp. 223-237). New York: National League for Nursing.

Allison, S., McLaughlin, K., & Walker, D. (1991). Nursing theory: A tool to put nursing back into nursing administration. *Nursing Administration Quarterly, 15*(3), 72-78.

Batey, M. V. (1977). Conceptualization: Knowledge and logic guiding empirical research. *Nursing Research, 26*(5), 324-329.

Bixler, G. K., & Bixler, R. W. (1959). The professional status of nursing. *American Journal of Nursing, 59*(8), 1142-1147.

Broncatello, K. F. (1980). Auger in action: Application of the model. *Advances in Nursing Science,* *3*(1), 13-23.

Carper, B. (1978). Fundamental patterns of knowing. *Advances in Nursing Science, 1*(1), 13-23.

Cross, P. (1981). *Adults as learners.* Washington, DC: Jossey-Bass.

Fawcett, J. (1978). The relationship between theory and research: A double helix. *Advances in Nursing Science, 1*(1), 49-62.

Fawcett, J. (1984). *Analysis and evaluation of conceptual models of nursing.* Philadelphia: F. A. Davis.

Fawcett, J. (1989). *Analysis and evaluation of conceptual models of nursing* (2nd ed.). Philadelphia: F. A. Davis.

Fawcett, J. (1995). *Analysis and evaluation of conceptual models of nursing* (3rd ed.). Philadelphia: F. A. Davis.

Field, P. A. (1987). The impact of nursing theory on the clinical decision making process. *Journal of Advanced Nursing, 12,* 563-571.

Huckabay, L. M. (1991). The role of conceptual frameworks in nursing practice, administration, education, and research. *Nursing Administration Quarterly, 15*(3), 17-28.

Johnson, D. E. (1968). Theory in nursing: Borrowed and unique. *Nursing Research, 17*(3), 206-209.

Johnson, D. E. (1974). Development of theory: A requisite for nursing as a primary health profession. *Nursing Research, 23*(5), 372-377.

Johnson, D. E. (1980). The behavioral system model for nursing. In J. P. Riehl & C. Roy (Eds.), *Conceptual models for nursing practice.* Norwalk, CT: Appleton-Century-Crofts.

Kalish, P. A., & Kalish, B. J. (1995). *The advance of American nursing* (3rd ed). Philadelphia: J. B. Lippincott.

King, I. (1971). *Toward a theory for nursing: General concepts of human behavior.* New York: John Wiley & Sons.

Kuhn, T. S. (1970). *The structure of scientific revolutions* (2nd ed.). Chicago: University of Chicago Press.

Levine, M. E. (1967). The four conservation principles of nursing. *Nursing Forum, 6,* 45-59.

Levine, M. E. (1995). The rhetoric of nursing theory. *IMAGE: Journal of Nursing Scholarship, 27*(1), 11-14.

Martin, M., Forchuk, C., Santopinto, M., & Butcher, H. K. (1992). Alternative approaches to nursing practice: Application of Peplau, Rogers, and Parse. *Nursing Science Quarterly, 5*(2), 80-85.

Mathwig, G. (1975). Translation of nursing science theory to nursing education. In S. Ketefian (Ed.), *Translation of theory into nursing practice and education.* Proceedings of the Seventh Annual Clinical Sessions, Continuing Education in Nursing Division of Nursing, School of Education, Health, Nursing, and Arts Professions, New York University.

Meleis, A. (1983). The evolving nursing scholars. In P. Chinn (Ed.), *Advances in nursing theory development.* Rockville, Md: Aspen.

Meleis, A. I. (1991). *Theoretical nursing: Development & progress* (2nd ed.). Philadelphia: J. B. Lippincott.

National League for Nursing (1992). *Criteria for evaluation of baccalaureate and higher degree programs in nursing* (7th ed.). New York: Author.

Neuman, B. (1972). A model for teaching total person approach to patient problems. *Nursing Research, 21*(3), 264-269.

Nicoll, L. H. (1986). *Perspectives on nursing theory.* Boston: Little, Brown.

Nurse Educator Conference (program), The First Annual (1977). *From student to effective professional.* Hyatt Regency, Chicago.

Nurse Educator Conference (program), The Second Annual (1978). *Nursing theory: Foundation for the future.* New York Hilton, New York City.

Oliver, N. R. (1991). True believers: A case for model-based nursing practice. *Nursing Administration Quarterly, 15*(3), 37-43.

Orem, D. E. (1971). *Nursing: Concepts of practice.* New York: McGraw-Hill.

Paul, R. W., & Nosich, G. M. (1991). *Proposal for the national assessment of higher-order thinking* (edited and revised version). The United States Department of Education Office of Educational Research and Improvement, National Center for Education Statistics.

Rogers, M. E. (1961). *Educational revolution in nursing.* New York: Macmillan.

Rogers, M. E. (1970). *An introduction to the theoretical basis of nursing.* Philadelphia: F. A. Davis.

Roy, C. (1970). Adaptation: A conceptual framework for nursing. *Nursing Outlook, 18*(3), 43-45.

Schlotfeldt, R. M. (1992). Why promote clinical nursing scholarship? *Clinical Nursing Research, 1*(1), 5-8.

Sparacino, P. (1991). The reciprocal relationship between practice and theory. *Clinical Nurse Specialist, 5*(3), 138.

Styles, M. M. (1982). *On nursing toward a new endowment.* St. Louis: Mosby.

Wardle, M. G., & Mandle, C. L. (1989). Conceptual models used in clinical practice. *Western Journal of Nursing Research, 11*(1), 108-114.

Whall, A. L. (1989). Nursing science: The process and the products. In J. J. Fitzpatrick, & A. L. Whall (Eds.), *Conceptual models of nursing* (pp. 1-14). Norwalk, CT: Appleton & Lange.

Models and Theories in Nursing Practice

Martha Raile Alligood

Nursing practice: "the acid test of nursing theory."
(Martin, Forchuk, Santopinto, & Butcher, 1992)

The use of models and theories in nursing practice is presented in this chapter, documenting various areas of application and utilization of the models as reported in the nursing literature. In line with the premise set forth in Chapter 1, the shift in emphasis from theory development to theory utilization restores a proper relationship between theory and practice for a professional discipline such as nursing. The importance of this shift is supported by Levine (1995), who noted in reference to Fawcett's clarification of models from theories, "It may be that the first prerequisite for effective use of theory in practice . . . rest[s] on just such a clarification" (p. 12). Nursing models and their theories have practical utility for nursing with details specific to practice in various areas.

This chapter presents the areas in which nursing models and their theories guide nursing practice based on a review of the nursing literature. Three tables present the use of the seven models in nursing practice (1) in terms of the medical model; (2) in terms of nursing based on human development, areas of practice, type of care, and type of health; and (3) in terms of nursing interventions. (See Bibliography for references to applications of each model cited in Tables 2-1, 2-2, and 2-3.)

It became apparent from the literature review that nurses describe their practice in several different ways. Some describe nursing practice in terms of the medical model, which focuses on the recipient or area of care as noted in Table 2-1. Examples of this focus are the nursing of cardiovascular patients or intensive care patients.

TABLE 2-1 Areas of Practice with Nursing Models Described in Terms of Medical Model Focus

Practice Areas	Johnson	King	Levine	Neuman	Orem	Rogers	Roy
Acute care						•	
Adolescent cancer							•
Adult diabetes		•			•		
AIDS management	•			•		•	•
Alzheimer's disease							•
Ambulatory care					•	•	
Anxiety		•			•		
Breast cancer							•
Burns			•				
Cancer		•			•	•	
Cancer pain management	•						
Cardiac disease		•			•		•
Cardiomyopathy							•
Chronic pain			•			•	
Cognitive impairment				•			
Congestive heart failure			•				
Critical care		•		•	•	•	•
Guillain-Barré syndrome					•		
Heart variations						•	
Hemodialysis	•				•		
Hypernatremia							•
Intensive care				•	•	•	•
Kawasaki disease							•
Leukemia							•
Long-term care			•		•		
Medical illness		•		•		•	
Menopause		•					
Neurofibromatosis		•					
Oncology	•				•	•	
Orthopedics		•		•			
Osteoporosis							•
Ostomy care					•		
Pediatric						•	
Perioperative			•		•		•
Polio survivors						•	
Postanesthesia							•
Postpartum							•
Posttrauma							•
Preoperative adults			•				
Preoperative anxiety		•			•		
Pressure ulcers			•				
Renal disease		•		•	•		
Rheumatoid arthritis					•		
Schizophrenia							•
Substance abuse					•	•	
Terminal illness						•	•
Ventilator patient							•
Ventricular tachycardia	•						
Wound healing			•				

TABLE 2-2 Areas of Practice with Nursing Models Based on Human Development, Type of Practice, Type of Care, or Type of Health Focus

Practice Areas	Johnson	King	Levine	Neuman	Orem	Rogers	Roy
Cesarean father							•
Child health		•					
Child psychiatric				•			
Dying process						•	
Emergency		•	•	•			•
Gerontology		•		•	•	•	•
High-risk infants		•					
Holistic care			•				
Homeless			•				
Hospice			•		•		
Managed care		•					
Mental health	•			•	•	•	
Neonates							•
Nursing administration		•		•	•	•	
Nursing adolescents	•	•			•		
Nursing adults		•	•	•	•	•	
Nursing children	•	•			•	•	•
Nursing community	•	•		•	•	•	•
Nursing elderly		•	•	•	•	•	•
Nursing families		•		•	•		
Nursing home residents						•	
Nursing infants			•		•		•
Nursing in space						•	
Nursing service						•	
Nursing women					•	•	
Occupational health					•		
Palliative care							•
Psychiatric nursing						•	
Public health				•			
Quality assurance	•						
Rehabilitation			•	•	•	•	•
Risk reduction				•			

Several observations are made about this focus (Table 2-1). First, it represents the largest body of literature. Second, each of the models is represented within this focus. Although this large grouping is surprising, in light of the efforts of the past 30 years to move nursing beyond the medical view to a nursing perspective, this focus reflects the practice area of the largest single group (68%) of practicing nurses, which according to the American Nurses Association's *Facts about Nursing* (1988) continues to be acute or illness care in hospitals.

Table 2-2 presents model and theory use in publications in which nurses describe their practice in terms of a developmental or life-span focus, nursing practice aimed at a particular group in society, a type of care, or a type of health. Examples of this focus are nursing of children, homeless, holistic care, or child health. Table 2-2 reflects the second largest group of articles. Like Table 2-1, Table 2-2 is represented by articles based on all seven of the nursing models included in this text. Although Table 2-2 is large, it represents a grouping of several different perspectives that continue to represent nursing thought: nursing of groups according to a developmental category, areas of practice, types of care, and types of health or health promotion.

Table 2-3 presents model and theory use in publications with a focus on a nursing intervention or the nursing role. Examples of this focus are life review and counseling. This table is smaller than Tables 2-1 and 2-2 and also differs in that not all of the nursing models are represented in Table 2-3. Certain nurses practicing from the perspective of nursing models seem to describe their practice in terms of a nursing intervention or nursing role. It is noted that the specificity of the language in Rogerian science has created several unique categories in this focus. This is not surprising considering the following. First, the development of a science calls for specific language. Second, a purpose of nursing science is to develop knowledge specific to the discipline perspective, so one would expect new intervention categories to be created rather than continuing to fit into other previously used categories. Third, one would expect the categories to be descriptive of the uniqueness of the nurse's perspective.

It is suggested that the nursing categories in Tables 2-2 and 2-3 may be considered in the context of Kuhn's discussion of normal science (1970).

TABLE 2-3 Areas of Model Use with a Nursing Intervention or Role Focus							
Practice Areas	**Johnson**	**King**	**Levine**	**Neuman**	**Orem**	**Rogers**	**Roy**
Breastfeeding				●			●
Community presence						●	
Counseling						●	
Family therapy		●		●			
Group therapy		●				●	●
Health patterning						●	
Imagery						●	
Intentionality						●	
Knowing participation						●	
Life-patterning difficulties						●	
Life review						●	
Nutrition				●			
Parenting		●		●			
Storytelling						●	
Therapeutic touch						●	

Paradigms (or nursing models) are not only frameworks to think about nursing but also structures that guide research and practice. As such, their use by members of the profession produces knowledge that guides practice as well as further research and theory development. Normal science gives evidence of the growing maturity of a discipline as it moves beyond an emphasis on knowledge development to knowledge use. Model-based nursing practice literature reflects growth toward normal science.

References

American Nurses Association. (1988). *Facts about nursing*. Kansas City: Author.

Kuhn, T. S. (1970). *The structure of scientific revolutions* (2nd ed.). Chicago: University of Chicago Press.

Martin M., Forchuk, C., Santopinto, M., & Butcher, H. (1992). Alternate approaches to nursing practice: Application of Peplau, Rogers, and Parse. *Nursing Science Quarterly, 5*(2), 80-85.

Bibliography
Johnson

Broncatello, K. F. (1980). Auger in action: Application of the model. *Advances in Nursing Science, 2*(2), 13-24.

Derdiarian, A. K. (1990). Comprehensive assessment of AIDS patients using the behavioral systems model for nursing practice instrument. *Journal of Advanced Nursing, 15*(4), 436-446.

Derdiarian, A. K. (1990). Effects of using systematic assessment instruments on patient and nurse satisfaction with nursing care. *Oncology Nursing Forum, 17*(1), 95-101.

Derdiarian, A. K. (1991). Effects of using a nursing model–based assessment instrument on quality of nursing care. *Journal of Nursing Administration, 15*(3), 1-16.

Fruehwirth, S. E. S. (1989). An application of Johnson's behavioral model: A case study. *Journal of Community Health Nursing, 6*(2), 61-71.

Herbert, J. (1989). A model for Anna. *Nursing, 3*(42), 30-34.

Holaday, B. (1987). Patterns of interaction between mothers and their chronically ill infants. *Maternal-Child Nursing Journal, 16*, 29-45.

McCauley, K., Choromanski, J. D., Wallinger, C., & Liu, K. (1984). Current management of ventricular tachycardia: Symposium from the Hospital of the University of Pennsylvania. Learning to live with controlled ventricular tachycardia: Utilizing the Johnson model. *Heart and Lung, 13*, 633-638.

Niemela, K., Poster, E. C., & Moreau, D. (1992). The attending nurse: A new role for the advanced clinician in an adolescent inpatient unit. *Journal of Child and Adolescent Psychiatric and Mental Health Nursing, 5*(3), 5-12.

Rawls, A. C. (1980). Evaluation of the Johnson behavioral model in clinical practice, *Image, 12*, 13-16.

Spratlen, L. P. (1976). Introducing ethnic-cultural factors in models of nursing: Some mental health applications. *Journal of Nursing Education, 15*(2), 23-29.

Wilkie, D. J. (1990). Cancer pain management: State of the art nursing care. *Nursing Clinics of North America, 25*(2), 331-343.

King

Alligood, M. R. (1995). Theory of goal attainment: Application to adult orthopedic nursing. In M. A. Frey & C. Sieloff (Eds.), *Advancing King's systems framework and theory of nursing* (pp. 209-222). Thousand Oaks, CA: Sage Publications.

Benedict, M., & Frey, M. (1995). Theory-based practice in the emergency department. In M. A. Frey, & C. Sieloff (Eds.), *Advancing King's systems framework and theory of nursing* (pp. 317-324). Thousand Oaks, CA: Sage Publications.

Davis, D. C. (1987). A conceptual framework for infertility. *Journal of Obstetric, Gynecologic, and Neonatal Nursing, 16,* 30-35.

DeHowitt, M. C. (1992). King's conceptual model and individual psychotherapy. *Perspectives in Psychiatric Care, 28*(4), 11-14.

Fawcett, J. M., Vaillancourt, V. M., & Watson, C. A. (1995). Integration of King's framework into nursing practice. In M. A. Frey & C. Sieloff (Eds.), *Advancing King's systems framework and theory of nursing* (pp. 176-191). Thousand Oaks, CA: Sage Publications.

Gonot, P. W. (1986). Family therapy as derived from King's conceptual model. In A. L. Whall (Ed.), *Family therapy theory for nursing: Four approaches* (pp. 33-48). Norwalk, CT: Appleton-Century-Crofts.

Hampton, D. C. (1994). King's theory of goal attainment as a framework for managed care implementation in a hospital setting. *Nursing Science Quarterly, 7*(4), 170-173.

Hanchett, E. S. (1990). Nursing models and community as client. *Nursing Science Quarterly, 3,* 67-72.

Hanna, K. M. (1995). Use of King's theory of goal attainment to promote adolescents' health behavior. In M. A. Frey & C. Sieloff (Eds.), *Advancing King's systems framework and theory of nursing* (pp. 239-250). Thousand Oaks, CA: Sage Publications.

Heggie, M., & Gangar, E. (1992). A nursing model for menopause clinics. *Nursing Standard, 6*(21), 32-34.

Hughes, M. M. (1983). Nursing theories and emergency nursing. *Journal of Emergency Nursing, 9,* 95-97.

Husband, A. (1988). Application of King's theory of nursing to the care of the adult with diabetes. *Journal of Advanced Nursing, 13*(4), 484-488.

Jolly, M. L., & Winker, C. K. (1995). Theory of goal attainment in the context of organizational structure. In M. A. Frey & C. Sieloff (Eds.), *Advancing King's systems framework and theory of nursing* (pp. 305-316). Thousand Oaks, CA: Sage Publications.

Jonas, C. M. (1987). King's goal attainment theory: Use in gerontological nursing practice. *Perspectives, 11*(4), 9-12.

Kenny, T. (1990). Erosion of individuality in care of elderly people in hospital—An alternative approach. *Journal of Advanced Nursing, 15,* 571-576.

King, I. M. (1983). The family coping with a medical illness: Analysis and application of King's theory of goal attainment. In I. W. Clements & F. B. Roberts (Eds.), *Family health: A theoretical approach to nursing care* (pp. 383-385). New York: John Wiley & Sons.

King, I. M. (1983). The family with an elderly member: Analysis and application of King's theory of goal attainment. In I. W. Clements & F. B. Roberts (Eds.), *Family health: A theoretical approach to nursing care* (pp. 341-345). New York: John Wiley & Sons.

King, I. M. (1984). Effectiveness of nursing care: Use of a goal-oriented nursing record in end-stage renal disease. *American Association of Nephrology Nurses and Technicians Journal, 11*(2), 11-17, 60.

Kohler, P. (1988). Model of shared control. *Journal of Gerontological Nursing, 14*(7), 21-25.

Laben, J. K., Dodd, D., & Sneed, L. D. (1991). King's theory of goal attainment applied in group therapy for inpatient juvenile sexual offenders, minimum security state offenders, and community parolees using visual aids. *Issues in Mental Health Nursing, 12*(1), 51-64.

Laben, J. K., Sneed, L. D., & Seidel, S. L. (1995). Goal attainment in short-term group psychotherapy settings. In M. A. Frey & C. Sieloff (Eds.), *Advancing King's systems framework and theory of nursing* (pp. 261-277). Thousand Oaks, CA: Sage Publications.

LaFontaine, P. (1989). Alleviating patient's apprehensions and anxieties. *Gastroenterology Nursing, 11,* 256-257.

Messmer, P. R. (1995). Implementation of theory-based nursing practice. In M. A. Frey & C. Sieloff (Eds.), *Advancing King's systems framework and theory of nursing* (pp. 294-304). Thousand Oaks, CA: Sage Publications.

Messner, R., & Smoth, M. N. (1986). Neurofibromatosis: Relinquishing the masks: A quest for quality of life. *Journal of Advanced Nursing, 11*, 459-464.

Norris, D. M., & Hoyer, P. J. (1993). Dynamism in practice: Parenting within King's framework. *Nursing Science Quarterly, 1*, 145-146.

Sirles, A. T., & Selleck, C. S. (1989). Cardiac disease and the family: Impact, assessment, and implications. *Journal of Cardiovascular Nursing, 3*(2), 23-32.

Smith, M. C. (1988). King's theory in practice. *Nursing Science Quarterly, 1*, 145-146.

Steele, S. (1981). *Child health and the family: Nursing concepts and management.* New York: Masson Publishing USA.

Swindale, J. E. (1989). The nurse's role in giving preoperative information to reduce anxiety in patients admitted to hospital for elective minor surgery. *Journal of Advanced Nursing, 14*, 899-905.

Symanski, M. E. (1991). Use of nursing theories in the care of families with high-risk infants: Challenges for the future. *Journal of Perinatal and Neonatal Nursing, 4*(4), 71-77.

Temple, A., & Fawdry, K. (1992). King's theory of goal attainment: Resolving filial caregiver role strain. *Journal of Gerontological Nursing, 18*(3), 11-15.

Woods, E. C. (1994). King's theory in practice with elders. *Nursing Science Quarterly, 7*(2), 65-69.

Levine

Bayley, E. W. (1991). Care of the burn patient. In K. M. Schaefer & J. A. B. Pond (Eds.), *Levine's conservation model: A framework for nursing practice* (pp. 91-99). Philadelphia: F. A. Davis.

Brunner, M. (1985). A conceptual approach to critical care using Levine's model. *Focus on Critical Care, 12*(2), 39-44.

Cooper, D. M. (1990). Optimizing wound healing: A practice within nursing's domain. *Nursing Clinics of North America, 25*, 165-180.

Cox, R. A. Sr. (1991). A tradition of caring: Use of Levine's model in long-term care. In K. M. Schaefer & J. A. B. Pond (Eds.), *Levine's conservation model: A framework for nursing practice* (pp. 179-197). Philadelphia: F. A. Davis.

Crawford-Gamble, P. E. (1986). An application of Levine's conceptual model. *Perioperative Nursing Quarterly, 2*(1), 64-70.

Dever, M. (1991). In K. M. Schaefer & J. A. B. Pond (Eds.), *Levine's conservation model: A framework for nursing practice* (pp. 71-82). Philadelphia: F. A. Davis.

Fawcett, J., Archer, C. L., Becker, D., Brown, K. K., Gann, S., Wong, M. J., & Wurster, A. B. (1992). Guidelines for selecting a conceptual model of nursing: Focus on the individual patient. *Dimensions of Critical Care Nursing, 11*, 268-277.

Fawcett, J., Cariello, F. P., Davis, D. A., Farley, J., Simmaro, D. M., & Watts, R. J. (1987). Conceptual models of nursing: Application to critical care nursing practice. *Dimensions of Critical Care Nursing, 6*, 202-213.

Hanson, D., Langemo, D. K., Olson, B., Hunter, S., Sauvage, T. R., Burd, C., & Cathcart-Silberberg, T. (1991). The prevalence and incidence of pressure ulcers in the hospice setting: Analysis of two methodologies. *American Journal of Hospice and Palliative Care, 8*(5), 18-22.

Herbst, S. (1981). Impairments as a result of cancer. In N. Martin, N. Holt, & D. Hicks (Eds.), *Comprehensive rehabilitation nursing* (pp. 553-578). New York: McGraw-Hill.

Pasco, A., & Halupa, D. (1991). Chronic pain management. In K. M. Schaefer & J. A. B. Pond (Eds.), *Levine's conservation model: A framework for nursing practice* (pp. 101-117). Philadelphia: F. A. Davis.

Pond, J. A. B. (1991). Ambulatory care of the homeless. In K. M. Schaefer & J. A. B. Pond (Eds.), *Levine's conservation model: A framework for nursing practice* (pp. 167-178). Philadelphia: F. A. Davis.

Pond, J. A. B., & Taney, S. G. (1991). Emergency care in a large university emergency department. In K. M. Schaefer & J. A. B. Pond (Eds.), *Levine's conservation model: A framework for nursing practice* (pp. 151-166). Philadelphia: F. A. Davis.

Savage, T. A., & Culbert, C. (1989). Early intervention: The unique role of nursing. *Journal of Pediatric Nursing, 4,* 339-345.

Schaefer, K. M. (1991). Care of the patient with congestive heart failure. In K. M. Schaefer & J. A. B. Pond (Eds.), *Levine's conservation model: A framework for nursing practice* (pp. 119-131). Philadelphia: F. A. Davis.

Schaefer, K. M., & Pond, J. A. B. (1994). Levine's conservation model as a guide to nursing practice. *Nursing Science Quarterly, 7*(2), 53-54.

Webb, H. (1993). Holistic care following a palliative Hartmann's procedure. *British Journal of Nursing, 2,* 128-132.

Neuman

Anderson, E., McFarlane, J., & Helton, A. (1986). Community-as-client: A model for practice. *Nursing Outlook, 34,* 220-224.

Baerg, K. L. (1991). Using Neuman's model to analyze a clinical situation. *Rehabilitation Nursing, 16,* 38-39.

Beckingham, A. C., & Baumann, A. (1990). The aging family in crisis: Assessment and decision-making models. *Journal of Advanced Nursing, 15,* 782-787.

Beddome, G. (1995). Community-as-client assessment. In B. Neuman (Ed.), *The Neuman systems model* (3rd ed., pp. 567-579). Norwalk, CT: Appleton & Lange.

Beitler, B., Tkachuck, B., & Aamodt, D. (1980). The Neuman model applied to mental health, community health, and medical-surgical nursing. In J. P. Riehl & C. Roy (Eds.), *Conceptual models for nursing practice* (2nd ed., pp. 170-178). New York: Appleton-Century-Crofts.

Bergstrom, D. (1992). Hypermetabolism in multisystem organ failure: A Neuman systems perspective. *Critical Care Nursing Quarterly, 15*(3), 63-70.

Biley, F. C. (1989). Stress in high dependency units. *Intensive Care Nursing, 5,* 134-141.

Breckenridge, D. M. (1995). Nephrology practice and directions for nursing research. In B. Neuman (Ed.), *The Neuman systems model* (3rd ed., pp. 499-507). Norwalk, CT: Appleton & Lange.

Brown, M. W. (1988). Neuman's systems model in risk factor reduction. *Cardiovascular Nursing, 24*(6), 43.

Buchanan, B. F. (1987). Human-environment interaction: A modification of the Neuman systems model for aggregates, families, and the community. *Public Health Nursing, 4,* 52-64.

Bueno, M. M., & Sengin, K. K. (1995). The Neuman systems model for critical care nursing. In B. Neuman (Ed.), *The Neuman systems model* (3rd ed., pp. 275-291). Norwalk, CT: Appleton & Lange.

Chiverton, P., & Flannery, J. C. (1995). Cognitive impairment. In B. Neuman (Ed.), *The Neuman systems model* (3rd ed., pp. 249-261). Norwalk, CT: Appleton & Lange.

Cunningham, S. G. (1983). The Neuman systems model applied to a rehabilitation setting. *Rehabilitation Nursing, 8*(4), 20-22.

Delunas, L. R. (1990). Prevention of elder abuse: Betty Neuman health care systems approach. *Clinical Nurse Specialist, 4,* 54-58.

Evely, L. (1994). A model for successful breastfeeding. *Modern Midwife, 4*(12), 25-27.

Fawcett, J., Archer, C. L., Becker, D., Brown, K. K., Gann, S., Wong, J. J., & Wurster, A. B. (1992). Guidelines for selecting a conceptual model of nursing: Focus on the individual patient. *Dimensions of Critical Care Nursing, 11,* 268-277.

Fawcett, J., Cariello, F. P., Davis, D. A., Farley, J., Simmaro, D. M., & Watts, R. J. (1987). Conceptual models of nursing: Application to critical care nursing practice. *Dimensions of Critical Care Nursing, 6,* 202-213.

Foote, A. W., Piazza, D., & Schultz, M. (1990). The Neuman systems model: Application to a patient with a cervical spinal cord injury. *Journal of Neuroscience Nursing, 22,* 302-306.

Fulbrook, P. R. (1991). The application of the Neuman systems model to intensive care. *Intensive Care Nursing, 7,* 28-39.

Galloway, D. A. (1993). Coping with a mentally and physically impaired infant: A self-analysis. *Rehabilitation Nursing, 18,* 34-36.

Gavan, C. A. S., Hastings-Tolsma, M. T., & Troyan, P. J. (1988). Explication of Neuman's model: A holistic systems approach to nutrition for health promotion in the life process. *Holistic Nursing Practice, 3*(1), 26-38.

Herrick, C. A., & Goodykoontz, L. (1989). Neuman's systems model for nursing practice as a conceptual framework for a family assessment. *Journal of Child and Adolescent Psychiatric and Mental Health Nursing, 2,* 61-67.

Herrick, C. A., Goodykoontz, L., Herrick, R. H., & Hackett, B. (1991). Planning a continuum of care in child psychiatric nursing: A collaborative effort. *Journal of Child and Adolescent Psychiatric and Mental Health Nursing, 4,* 41-48.

Hiltz, D. (1990). The Neuman systems model: An analysis of a clinical situation. *Rehabilitation Nursing, 15,* 330-332.

Hoeman, S. P., & Winters, D. M. (1990). Theory-based case management: High cervical spinal cord injury. *Home Healthcare Nurse, 8,* 25-33.

Kelly, J. S., & Sanders, N. F. (1995). A systems approach to the health of nursing and health care organizations. In B. Neuman (Ed.), *The Neuman systems model* (3rd ed., pp. 347-364). Norwalk, CT: Appleton & Lange.

Kido, L. M. (1991). Sleep deprivation and intensive care unit psychosis. *Emphasis: Nursing, 4*(1), 23-33.

Knight, J. B. (1990). The Betty Neuman systems model applied to practice: A client with multiple sclerosis. *Journal of Advanced Nursing, 15,* 447-455.

Lindell, M., & Olsson, H. (1991). Can combined oral contraceptives be made more effective by means of a nursing care model? *Journal of Advanced Nursing, 16,* 475-479.

Millard, J. (1992). Health visiting an elderly couple. *British Journal of Nursing, 1,* 769-773.

Miner, J. (1995). Incorporating the Betty Neuman systems model into HIV clinical practice. *AIDS Patient Care, 9*(1), 37-39.

Moore, S. L., & Munro, M. F. (1990). The Neuman systems model applied to mental health nursing of older adults. *Journal of Advanced Nursing, 15,* 293-299.

Piazza, D., Foote, A., Wright, P., & Holcombe, J. (1992). Neuman systems model used as a guide for the nursing care of an 8-year-old child with leukemia. *Journal of Pediatric Oncology Nursing, 9*(1), 17-24.

Pierce, A. G., & Gulmer, T. T. (1995). Application of the Neuman systems model to gerontological nursing. In B. Neuman (Ed.), *The Neuman systems model* (3rd ed., pp. 293-308). Norwalk, CT: Appleton & Lange.

Pierce, J. D., & Hutton, E. (1992). Applying the new concepts of the Neuman systems model. *Nursing Forum, 27,* 15-18.

Redheffer, G. (1985). Application of Betty Neuman's health care systems model to emergency nursing practice: Case review. *Point of View, 22*(2), 4-6.

Reed, K. S. (1993). Adapting the Neuman systems model for family nursing. *Nursing Science Quarterly, 6,* 93-97.

Ross, M., & Bourbonnais, F. (1985). The Betty Neuman systems model in nursing practice: A case study approach. *Journal of Advanced Nursing, 10,* 199-207.

Ross, M., & Helmer, H. (1988). A comparative analysis of Neuman's model using the individual and family as the units of care. *Public Health Nursing, 5,* 30-36.

Russell, J., Hileman, J. W., & Grant, J. S. (1995). Assessing and meeting the needs of home caregivers using the Neuman systems model. In B. Neuman (Ed.), *The Neuman systems model* (3rd ed., pp. 331-341). Norwalk, CT: Appleton & Lange.

Shaw, M. C. (1991). A theoretical base for orthopaedic nursing practice: The Neuman systems model. *Canadian Orthopaedic Nurses Association Journal, 13*(2), 19-21.

Smith, M. C. (1989). Neuman's model in practice. *Nursing Science Quarterly, 1,* 116-117.

Sohier, R. (1995). Nursing care for the people of a small planet: Culture and the Neuman systems model. In B. Neuman (Ed.), *The Neuman systems model* (3rd ed., pp. 101-117). Norwalk, CT: Appleton & Lange.

Stuart, G., & Wright, L. K. (1995). In B. Neuman (Ed.), *The Neuman systems model* (3rd ed., pp. 263-273). Norwalk, CT: Appleton & Lange.

Sullivan, J. (1986). Using Neuman's model in the acute phase of spinal cord injury. *Focus on Critical Care, 13*(5), 34-41.

Trepanier, M. J., Dunn, S. I., & Sprague, A. E. (1995). Application of the Neuman systems model to perinatal nursing. In B. Neuman (Ed.), *The Neuman systems model* (3rd ed., pp. 309-320). Norwalk, CT: Appleton & Lange.

Utz, S. W. (1980). Applying the Neuman model to nursing practice with hypertensive clients. *Cardiovascular Nursing, 16,* 29-34.

Wallingford, P. (1989). The neurologically impaired and dying child: Applying the Neuman systems model. *Issues in Comprehensive Pediatric Nursing, 12,* 139-157.

Ware, L. A., & Shannahan, M. D. (1995). Using Neuman for a stable parent support group in neonatal intensive care. In B. Neuman (Ed.), *The Neuman systems model* (3rd ed., pp. 321-330). Norwalk, CT: Appleton & Lange.

Weinberger, S. L. (1991). Analysis of a clinical situation using the Neuman system model. *Rehabilitation Nursing, 16,* 278, 280-281.

Orem

Anderson, S. B. (1992). Guillain-Barré syndrome: Giving the patient control. *Journal of Neuroscience Nursing, 24,* 158-162.

Atkins, F. D. (1992). An uncertain future: Children of mentally ill parents. *Journal of Psychosocial Nursing and Mental Health Services, 30*(8), 13-16.

Beckmann, C. A. (1987). Maternal-child health in Brazil. *Journal of Obstetric, Gynecologic, and Neonatal Nursing, 16,* 238-241.

Berbiglia, V. A. (1991). A case study: Perspectives on a self-care deficit nursing theory–based curriculum. *Journal of Advanced Nursing, 16,* 1158-1163.

Blaylock, B. (1991). Enhancing self-care of the elderly client: Practical teaching tips for ostomy care. *Journal of Enterostomal Therapy Nursing, 18,* 118-121.

Buckwalter, K. C., & Kerfoot, K. M. (1982). Teaching patients self-care: A critical aspect of psychiatric discharge planning. *Journal of Psychiatric Nursing and Mental Health Services, 20*(5), 15-20.

Campuzano, M. (1982). Self-care following coronary artery bypass surgery. *Focus on Critical Care, 9*(2), 55-56.

Cantanese, M. L. (1987). Vaginal birth after cesarean: Recommendations, risks, realities, and the client's right to know. *Holistic Nursing Practice, 2*(1), 35-43.

Caradus, A. (1991). Nursing theory and operating suite nursing practice. *ACORN Journal, 4*(2), 29-30, 32.

Clark, M. D. (1986). Application of Orem's theory of self-care: A case study. *Journal of Community Health Nursing, 3*(3), 127-135.

Comptom, P. (1989). Drug abuse: A self-care deficit. *Journal of Psychosocial Nursing and Mental Health Services, 27*(3), 22-26.

Connelly, C. E. (1987). Self-care and the chronically ill patient. *Nursing Clinics of North America, 22,* 621-629.

Cretain, G. K. (1989). Motivational factors in breast self-examination: Implications for nurses. *Cancer Nursing, 12,* 250-256.

Davidhizar, R., & Cosgray, R. (1990). The use of Orem's model in psychiatric rehabilitation assessment. *Rehabilitation Nursing, 15*(1), 39-41.

Dear, M. R., & Keen, M. F. (1982). Promotion of self-care in the employee with rheumatoid arthritis. *Occupational Health Nursing, 30*(1), 32-34.

Dropkin, M. J. (1981). Development of a self-care teaching program for postoperative head and neck patients. *Cancer Nursing, 4,* 103-106.

Duffy, J., Miller, M. P., & Parlocha, P. (1993). Psychiatric home care: A framework for assessment and intervention. *Home Healthcare Nurse, 11*(2), 22-28.

Dunn, B. (1990). Alcohol dependency: Health promotion and Orem's model. *Nursing Standard, 4*(40), 34.

Eichelberger, K. M., Kaufman, D. N., Rundahl, M. E., & Schwartz, N. E. (1980). Self-care nursing plan: Helping children to help themselves. *Pediatric Nursing, 6*(3), 9-13.

Eliopoulos, C. (1984). A self-care model for gerontological nursing. *Geriatric Nursing, 4,* 366-369.

Facteau, L. M. (1980). Self-care concepts and the care of the hospitalized child. *Nursing Clinics of North America, 15,* 145-155.

Fawcett, J., Archer, C. L., Becker, D., Brown, K. K., Gann, S., Wong, J. J., & Wurster, A. B. (1992). Guidelines for selecting a conceptual model of nursing: Focus on the individual patient. *Dimensions of Critical Care Nursing, 11,* 268-277.

Fawcett, J., Cariello, F. P., Davis, D. A., Farley, J., Simmaro, D. M., & Watts, R. J. (1987). Conceptual models of nursing: Application to critical care nursing practice. *Dimensions of Critical Care Nursing, 6*(4), 202-213.

Fields, L. M. (1987). A clinical application of the Orem nursing model in labor and delivery. *Emphasis: Nursing, 2,* 102-108.

Fitzgerald, S. (1980). Utilizing Orem's self-care model in designing an education program for the diabetic. *Topics in Clinical Nursing, 2*(2), 57-65.

Flanagan, M. (1991). Self-care for a leg ulcer. *Nursing Times, 87*(23), 67-68, 70, 72.

Foote, A., Holcombe, J., Piazza, D., & Wright, P. (1993). Orem's theory used as a guide for the nursing care of an eight-year-old child with leukemia. *Journal of Pediatric Oncology Nursing, 10*(1), 26-32.

Fridgen, R., & Nelson, S. (1992). Teaching tool for renal transplant recipients using Orem's self-care model. *CANNT, 2*(3), 18-26.

Geyer, E. (1990). Self-care issues for the elderly. *Dimensions in Oncology Nursing, 4*(2), 33-35.

Haas, D. L. (1990). Application of Orem's self-care deficit theory to the pediatric chronically ill population. *Issues in Comprehensive Pediatric Nursing, 13,* 253-264.

Hanchett, E. S. (1990). Nursing models and community as client. *Nursing Science Quarterly, 3,* 67-72.

Harris, J. K. (1980). Self-care is possible after cesarean delivery. *Nursing Clinics of North America, 15,* 191-204.

Hurst, J. D., & Stullenbarger, B. (1986). Implementation of a self-care approach in a pediatric interdisciplinary phenylketonuria (PKU) clinic. *Journal of Pediatric Nursing, l,* 159-163.

Jacobs, C. J. (1990). Orem's self-care model: Is it relevant to patients in intensive care? *Intensive Care Nursing, 6,* 100-103.

Kam, B. W., & Werner, P. W. (1990). Self-care theory: Application to perioperative nursing. *Association of Operating Room Nurses Journal, 51,* 1365-1370.

Keohane, N. S., & Lacey, L. A. (1991). Preparing the woman with gestational diabetes for self-care: Use of a structured teaching plan for nursing staff. *Journal of Obstetric, Gynecologic, and Neonatal Nursing, 20,* 189-193.

Komulainen, P. (1991). Occupational health nursing based on self-care theory. *American Association of Occupational Health Nursing Journal, 39,* 333-335.

Kyle, B. A. S., & Pitzer, S. A. (1990). A self-care approach to today's challenges. *Nursing Management, 21*(3), 37-39.

Lacey, D. (1993). Using Orem's model in psychiatric nursing. *Nursing Standard, 7*(29), 28-30.

Mack, C. H. (1992). Assessment of the autologous bone marrow transplant patient according to Orem's self-care model. *Cancer Nursing, 15,* 429-436.

Meriney, D. K. (1990). Application of Orem's conceptual framework to patients with hypercalcemia related to breast cancer. *Cancer Nursing, 13,* 316-323.

Morse, W., & Werner, J. S. (1988). Individualization of patient care using Orem's theory. *Cancer Nursing, 11,* 195-202.

Moscovitz, A. (1984). Orem's theory as applied to psychiatric nursing. *Perspectives in Psychiatric Care, 22*(1), 36-38.

Mullin, V. I. (1980). Implementing the self-care concept in the acute care setting. *Nursing Clinics of North America, 15,* 177-190.

Murphy, P. P. (1981). A hospice model and self-care theory. *Oncology Nursing Forum, 8*(2), 19-21.

Norris, M. K. G. (1991). Applying Orem's theory to the long-term care of adolescent transplant recipients. *American Nephrology Nurses' Association Journal, 18,* 45-47, 53.

O'Donovan, S. (1990). Nursing models: More of Orem. *Nursing the Elderly, 2*(3), 22-23.

O'Donovan, S. (1990). Nursing models: More of Orem. *Nursing the Elderly, 2*(4), 20-22.

Padula, C. A. (1992). Self-care and the elderly: Review and implications. *Public Health Nursing, 9,* 22-28.

Park, P. B. (1989). Health care for the homeless: A self-care approach. *Clinical Nurse Specialist, 3,* 171-175.

Perras, S., & Zappacosta, A. (1982). The application of Orem's theory in promoting self-care in a peritoneal dialysis facility. *American Association of Nephrology Nurses and Technicians Journal, 9*(3), 37-39.

Raven, M. (1988-1989). Application of Orem's self-care model to nursing practice in developmental disability. *Australian Journal of Advanced Nursing, 6*(2), 16-23.

Rew, L. (1990). Childhood sexual abuse: Toward a self-care framework for nursing intervention and research. *Archives of Psychiatric Nursing, 4,* 147-153.

Richardson, A. (1991). Theories of self-care: Their relevance to chemotherapy-induced nausea and vomiting. *Journal of Advanced Nursing, 16,* 671-676.

Smith, M. C. (1977). Self-care: A conceptual framework for rehabilitation nursing. *Rehabilitation Nursing, 2*(2), 8-10.

Smith, M. C. (1989). An application of Orem's theory in nursing practice. *Nursing Science Quarterly, 2*(4), 159-161.

Swindale, J. E. (1989). The nurse's role in giving preoperative information to reduce anxiety in patients admitted to hospital for elective minor surgery. *Journal of Advanced Nursing, 14,* 899-905.

Taylor, S. G. (1988). Nursing theory and nursing process: Orem's theory in practice. *Nursing Science Quarterly, 1,* 111-119.

Taylor, S. G. (1989). An interpretation of family with Orem's general theory of nursing. *Nursing Science Quarterly, 1,* 131-137.

Taylor, S. G. (1990). Practical applications of Orem's self-care deficit nursing theory. In M. E. Parker (Ed.), *Nursing theories in practice* (pp. 61-70). New York: National League for Nursing.

Taylor, S. G., & McLaughlin, K. (1991). Orem's general theory of nursing and community nursing. *Nursing Science Quarterly, 4,* 153-160.

Titus, S., & Porter, P. (1989). Orem's theory applied to pediatric residential treatment, *Pediatric Nursing, 15,* 465-468, 556.

Tolentino, M. B. (1990). The use of Orem's self-care model in the neonatal intensive care unit. *Journal of Obstetric, Gynecologic, and Neonatal Nursing, 19,* 496-500.

Vasquez, M. A. (1992). From theory to practice: Orem's self-care nursing model and ambulatory care. *Journal of Post Anesthesia Nursing, 7,* 251-255.

Walborn, K. A. (1980). A nursing model for the hospice: Primary and self-care nursing. *Nursing Clinics of North America, 15,* 205-217.

Walsh, M., & Judd, M. (1989). Long term immobility and self-care: The Orem nursing approach. *Nursing Standard, 3*(41), 34-36.

Zach, P. (1982). Self-care agency in diabetic ocular sequelae. *Journal of Ophthalmic Nursing Techniques, 1*(2), 21-31.

Rogers

Alligood, M. R. (1989). Rogers' theory and nursing administration: A perspective on health and environment. In B. Henry, C. Arndt, M. DiVincenti, & A. Marriner-Tomey (Eds.), *Dimensions of nursing administration: Theory, research, education, and practice* (pp. 105-111). Boston: Blackwell Scientific.

Alligood, M. R. (1990). Nursing care of the elderly: Futuristic projections. In E. A. M. Barrett (Ed.), *Visions of Rogers' science-based nursing* (pp. 129-142). New York: National League for Nursing.

Alligood, M. R. (1994). Toward a unitary view of nursing practice. In M. Madrid & E. A. M. Barrett (Eds.), *Rogers' scientific art of nursing practice* (pp. 223-237). New York: National League for Nursing.

Anderson, M. D., & Smereck, G. A. D. (1994). Personalized nursing: A science-based model of the art of nursing. In M. Madrid & E. A. M. Barrett (Eds.), *Rogers' scientific art of nursing practice* (pp. 261-283). New York: National League for Nursing.

Barrett, E. A. M. (1988). Using Rogers' science of unitary human beings in nursing practice. *Nursing Science Quarterly, 1,* 50-51.

Barrett, E. A. M. (1990). Health patterning in clients in a private practice. In E. A. M. Barrett (Ed.), *Visions of Rogers' science-based nursing* (pp. 105-116). New York: National League for Nursing.

Barrett, E. A. M. (1990). Rogers' science-based nursing practice. In E. A. M. Barrett (Ed.), *Visions of Rogers' science-based nursing* (pp. 31-44). New York: National League for Nursing.

Barrett, E. A. M. (1992). Innovative imagery: A health patterning modality for nursing practice. *Journal of Holistic Nursing, 10,* 154-166.

Barrett, E. A. M. (1993). Virtual reality: A health patterning modality for nursing in space. *Visions: The Journal of Rogerian Nursing Science, 1,* 10-21.

Black, G., & Haight, B. K. (1992). Integrality as a holistic framework for the life-review process. *Holistic Nursing Practice, 7*(1), 7-15.

Buczny, B., Speirs, J., & Howard, J. R. (1989). Nursing care of a terminally ill client. Applying Martha Rogers' conceptual framework. *Home Healthcare Nurse, 7*(4), 13-18.

Caroselli, C. (1994). Opportunities for knowing participation: A new design for the nursing service organization. In M. Madrid & E. A. M. Barrett (Eds.), *Rogers' scientific art of nursing practice* (pp. 243-259). New York: National League for Nursing.

Chapman, J. S., Mitchell, G. J., & Forchuk, C. (1994). A glimpse of nursing theory–based practice in Canada. *Nursing Science Quarterly, 7,* 104-112.

Christensen, P., Sowell, R., & Gueldner, S. H. (1993). Nursing in space: Theoretical foundations and potential practice applications within Rogerian science. *Visions: The Journal of Rogerian Nursing Science, 1,* 36-44.

Clarke, P. (1994). Nursing theory–based practice in the home and the community. *Advances in Nursing Science, 17*(2), 41-53.

Cowling, W. R. III. (1990). A template for unitary pattern-based nursing practice. In E. A. M. Barrett (Ed.), *Visions of Rogers' science-based nursing* (pp. 45-66). New York: National League for Nursing.

Forker, J. E., & Billings, C. V. (1989). Nursing therapeutics in a group encounter. *Archives of Psychiatric Nursing, 3,* 108-112.

France, N. E. M. (1994). Unitary human football players. In M. Madrid & E. A. M. Barrett (Eds.), *Rogers' scientific art of nursing practice* (pp. 197-206). New York: National League for Nursing.

Griffin, J. (1994). Storytelling as a scientific art form. In M. Madrid & E. A. M. Barrett (Eds.), *Rogers' scientific art of nursing practice* (pp. 101-104). New York: National League for Nursing.

Gueldner, S. H. (1994). Pattern diversity and community presence in the human-environmental process: Implications for Rogerian-based practice with nursing home residents. In M. Madrid & E. A. M. Barrett (Eds.), *Rogers' scientific art of nursing practice* (pp. 131-140). New York: National League for Nursing.

Hanchett, E. S. (1990). Nursing models and community as client. *Nursing Science Quarterly, 3,* 67-72.

Heggie, J., Garon, M., Kodiath, M., & Kelly, A. (1994). Implementing the science of unitary human beings at the San Diego Veterans Affairs Medical Center. In M. Madrid & E. A. M. Barrett (Eds.), *Rogers' scientific art of nursing practice* (pp. 285-304). New York: National League for Nursing.

Heggie, J. R., Schoenmehl, P. A., Chang, M. K., & Crieco, C. (1989). Selection and implementation of Dr. Martha Rogers' nursing conceptual model in an acute care setting. *Clinical Nurse Specialist, 3,* 143-147.

Hill, L., & Oliver, N. (1993). Technique integration: Therapeutic touch and theory-based mental health nursing. *Journal of Psychosocial Nursing and Mental Health Services, 31*(2), 19-22.

Horvath, B. (1994). The science of unitary human beings as a foundation for nursing practice with persons experiencing life patterning difficulties: Transforming theory into motion. In M. Madrid & E. A. M. Barrett (Eds.), *Rogers' scientific art of nursing practice* (pp. 163-176). New York: National League for Nursing.

Johnson, R. L. (1986). Approaching family intervention through Rogers' conceptual model. In A. L. Whall (Ed.), *Family therapy theory for nursing: Four approaches* (pp. 11-32). Norwalk, CT: Appleton-Century-Crofts.

Joseph, L. (1990). Practical application of Rogers' theoretical framework for nursing. In M. E. Parker (Ed.), *Nursing theories in practice* (pp. 115-125). New York: National League for Nursing.

Jurgens, A., Meehan, T. C., & Wilson, H. L. (1987). Therapeutic touch as a nursing intervention. *Holistic Nursing Practice, 2*(1), 1-13.

Kodiath, M. F. (1991). A new view of the chronic pain client. *Holistic Nursing Practice, 6*(1), 41-46.

Madrid, M. (1990). The participating process of human field patterning in an acute-care environment. In E. A. M. Barrett (Ed.), *Visions of Rogers' science-based nursing* (pp. 93-104). New York: National League for Nursing.

Madrid, M. (1994). Participating in the process of dying. In M. Madrid & E. A. M. Barrett (Eds.), *Rogers' scientific art of nursing practice* (pp. 91-100). New York: National League for Nursing.

Magan, S. J., Gibbon, E. J., & Mrozek, R. (1990). Nursing theory applications: A practice model. *Issues in Mental Health Nursing, 11,* 297-312.

Malinski, V. M. (1986). Nursing practice within the science of unitary human beings. In V. M. Malinski (Ed.), *Explorations on Martha Rogers' science of unitary human beings* (pp. 25-32). Norwalk, CT: Appleton-Century-Crofts.

Malinski, V. M. (1994). Health patterning for individuals and families. In M. Madrid & E. A. M. Barrett (Eds.), *Rogers' scientific art of nursing practice* (pp. 105-117). New York: National League for Nursing.

Meehan, T. C. (1990). The science of unitary human beings and theory-based practice: Therapeutic touch. In E. A. M. Barrett (Ed.), *Visions of Rogers' science-based nursing* (pp. 67-82. New York: National League for Nursing.

Morwessel, N. J. (1994). Developing an effective pattern appraisal to guide nursing of children with heart variations and their families. In M. Madrid & E. A. M. Barrett (Eds.), *Rogers' scientific art of nursing practice* (pp. 147-161). New York: National League for Nursing.

Newshan, G. (1989). Therapeutic touch for symptom control in person with AIDS. *Holistic Nursing Practice, 3*(4), 45-51.

Payne, M. B. (1989). The use of therapeutic touch with rehabilitation clients. *Rehabilitation Nursing, 14*(2), 69-72.

Sargent, S. (1994). Healing groups: Awareness of a group field. In M. Madrid & E. A. M. Barrett (Eds.), *Rogers' scientific art of nursing practice* (pp. 119-129). New York: National League for Nursing.

Smith, D. W. (1994). Viewing polio survivors through violet-tinted glasses. In M. Madrid & E. A. M. Barrett (Eds.), *Rogers' scientific art of nursing practice* (pp. 141-145). New York: National League for Nursing.

Thomas, S. D. (1990). Intentionality in the human-environment encounter in an ambulatory care environment. In E. A. M. Barrett (Ed.), *Visions of Rogers' science-based nursing* (pp. 117-128). New York: National League for Nursing.

Thompson, J. E. (1990). Finding the borderline's border: Can Martha Rogers help? *Perspectives in Psychiatric Care, 26*(4), 7-10.

Tudor, C. A., Keegan-Jones, L., & Bens, E. M. (1994). Implementing Rogers' science-based nursing practice in a pediatric nursing service setting. In M. Madrid & E. A. M. Barrett (Eds.), *Rogers' scientific art of nursing practice* (pp. 305-322). New York: National League for Nursing.

Tuyn, L. K. (1992). Solution-oriented therapy and Rogerian nursing science: An integrated approach. *Archives of Psychiatric Nursing, 6,* 83-89.

Tuyn, L. K. (1994). Rhythms of living: A Rogerian approach to counseling. In M. Madrid & E. A. M. Barrett (Eds.), *Rogers' scientific art of nursing practice* (pp. 207-221). New York: National League for Nursing.

Whall, A. (1981). Nursing theory and the assessment of families. *Journal of Psychiatric Nursing and Mental Health Services, 19*(1), 30-36.

Roy

Aaronson, L., & Seaman, L. P. (1989). Managing hypernatremia in fluid-deficient elderly. *Journal of Gerontological Nursing, 15*(7), 29-34.

Barnfather, J. S., Swain, M. A. P., & Erickson, H. C. (1989). Evaluation of two assessment techniques for adaptation to stress. *Nursing Science Quarterly, 2,* 172-182.

Bawden, M., Ralph, J., Herrick, C. A. (1991). Enhancing the coping skills of mothers with developmentally delayed children. *Journal of Child and Adolescent Psychiatric Mental Health Nursing, 4,* 25-28.

Caradus, A. (1991). Nursing theory and operating suite nursing practice. *ACORN Journal, 4*(2), 29-30, 32.

DiMaria, R. A. (1989). Posttrauma responses: Potential for nursing. *Journal of Advanced Medical-Surgical Nursing, 2*(1), 41-48.

Doyle, R., & Rajacich, D. (1991). The Roy adaptation model: Health teaching about osteoporosis. *American Association of Occupational Health Nursing Journal, 39,* 508-512.

Ellis, J. A. (1991). Coping with adolescent cancer: It's a matter of adaptation. *Journal of Pediatric Oncology Nursing, 8,* 10-17.

Fawcett, J. (1981). Assessing and understanding the cesarean father. In C. F. Kehoe (Ed.), *The cesarean experience: Theoretical and clinical perspectives for nurses* (pp. 143-156). New York: Appleton-Century-Crofts.

Fawcett, J., Archer, C. L., Becker, D., Brown, K. K., Gann, S., Wong, M. J., & Wurster, A. B. (1992). Guidelines for selecting a conceptual model of nursing: Focus on the individual patient. *Dimensions of Critical Care Nursing, 11,* 268-277.

Galligan, A. C. (1979). Using Roy's concept of adaptation to care for young children. *American Journal of Maternal Child Nursing, 4,* 24-28.

Gerrish, C. (1989). From theory to practice. *Nursing Times, 85*(35), 42-45.

Giger, J. A., Bower, C. A., & Miller, S. W. (1987). Roy adaptation model: ICU application. *Dimensions of Critical Care Nursing, 6,* 215-224.

Hamner, J. B. (1989). Applying the Roy adaptation model to the CCU. *Critical Care Nurse, 9*(3), 51-61.

Hanchett, E. S. (1990). Nursing models and community as client. *Nursing Science Quarterly, 3,* 67-72.

Hughes, M. M. (1983). Nursing theories and emergency nursing. *Journal of Emergency Nursing, 9,* 95-97.

Innes, M. H. (1992). Management of an inadequately ventilated patient. *British Journal of Nursing, 1,* 780-784.

Jackson, D. A. (1990). Roy in the postanesthesia care unit. *Journal of Post Anesthesia Nursing, 5,* 143-148.

Janelli, L. (1980). Utilizing Roy's adaptation model from a gerontological perspective. *Journal of Gerontological Nursing, 6,* 140-150.

Kehoe, C. F. (1981). Identifying the nursing needs of the postpartum cesarean mother. In C. F. Kehoe (Ed.), *The cesarean experience: Theoretical and clinical perspectives for nurses* (pp. 143-156). New York: Appleton-Century-Crofts.

Kurek-Ovshinsky, C. (1991). Group psychotherapy in an acute inpatient setting: Techniques that nourish self-esteem. *Issues in Mental Health Nursing, 12,* 81-88.

Logan, M. (1986). Palliative care nursing: Applicability of the Roy model. *Journal of Palliative Care, 1*(2), 18-24.

Logan, M. (1988). Care of the terminally ill includes the family. *The Canadian Nurse, 84*(5), 30-33.

McIver, M. (1987). Putting theory into practice. *The Canadian Nurse, 83*(10), 36-38.

Miller, F. (1991). Using Roy's model in a special hospital. *Nursing Standard, 5*(27), 29-32.

Nash, D. J. (1987). Kawasaki disease: Application of the Roy adaptation model to determine interventions. *Journal of Pediatric Nursing, 2,* 308-315.

Nyquist, K. H. (1993). Advice concerning breastfeeding from mothers of infants admitted to a neonatal intensive care unit: The Roy adaptation model as a conceptual structure. *Journal of Advanced Nursing, 18*(1), 54-63.

Piazza, D., & Foote, A. (1990). Roy's adaptation model: A guide for rehabilitation nursing practice. *Rehabilitation Nursing, 15,* 254-259.

Piazza, D., Foote, A., Holcombe, J., Harris, M. G., & Wright, P. (1992). The use of Roy's adaptation model applied to a patient with breast cancer. *European Journal of Cancer Care,1*(4), 17-22.

Schmidt, C. S. (1981). Withdrawal behavior of schizophrenics: Application of Roy's model. *Journal of Psychosocial Nursing and Mental Health Services, 19*(11), 26-33.

Sirignano, R. G. (1987). Peripartum cardiomyopathy: An application of the Roy adaptation model. *Journal of Cardiovascular Nursing, 2,* 24-32.

Smith, M. C. (1988). Roy's adaptation model in practice. *Nursing Science Quarterly, 1,* 97-98.

Thornbury, J. M., & King, L. D. (1992). The Roy adaptation model and care of persons with Alzheimer's disease. *Nursing Science Quarterly, 5,* 129-133.

Vavaro, F. F. (1991). Women with coronary heart disease: An application of Roy's adaptation model. *Cardiovascular Nursing, 27*(6), 31-35.

Weiss, M. E., Hastings, W. J., Holly, D. C., & Craig, D. I. (1994). Using Roy's adaptation model in practice: Nurses' perspectives. *Nursing Science Quarterly, 7,* 80-86.

Wright, P. S., Holcombe, J., Foote, A., & Piazza, D. (1993). The Roy adaptation model used as a guide for the nursing care of an 8-year-old child with leukemia. *Journal of Pediatric Oncology Nursing, 10,* 68-74.

Models and Theories: Critical Thinking Structures

Martha Raile Alligood

"It is not simply knowing a lot of things, it is a way of knowing things." (Levine, 1988)

Application of nursing theory in practice depends on nurses having knowledge of the models and theories as well as an understanding of how these models and theories relate to each other. Nursing theory has been clarified as less abstract than nursing models by Fawcett (1993, 1995), but what does that mean for the practicing nurse? This chapter answers that question by describing the relationship of each of the seven nursing models included in this text with their theories. Based on the patterns of knowing in nursing (Carper, 1978), the models and their theories represent the empirical pattern or the science of nursing. They are organizing frameworks for substantive approaches to nursing. They provide critical thinking structures to guide the reasoning of professional nursing practice. The basis for models as critical thinking structures is presented using the definition and process of critical thinking according to Paul and Nosich (1991). The chapter concludes with points to be considered when selecting a nursing model to guide practice. The importance of the fit between the nurse and the model is discussed. The reader who wishes to review the nursing models included in this text is referred to Unit III of *Nursing Theorists and their Work* (Marriner-Tomey, 1994, pp. 181-322) for analyses and critiques of the seven nursing models.

RELATIONSHIP OF NURSING MODELS AND THEORIES

The models of a discipline are frameworks or paradigms that address the central concepts of that discipline. The science of nursing is recognized as a fundamental pattern of knowing for nurses (Carper, 1978). A structure for that science has been proposed by Fawcett (1993, 1995) according to Kuhn's philosophy of science and scientific development (1970). This structure provides a context to understand the interrelationship of the elements of the science (Fawcett, 1989, 1993, 1995). Nursing models are the frameworks or paradigms of the science of nursing that address the person, environment, health, and nursing metaparadigm. Nursing theories that are derived from models are guiding structures for reasoning about the person as well as determinants of nursing action. Therefore a model is a structure for critical thinking, reasoning, and decision making in practice that provides a perspective of the person for whom the nurse cares and specifies the approach to be taken in the delivery of that care.

Models are broad conceptual structures that provide a total perspective of the phenomena of a discipline. What this means in terms of nursing practice is that the way nurses think about people and about nursing has a direct impact on how people are approached, what questions are asked, how information is learned and processed, and what nursing activities are included in nursing care.

Theories are also sets of concepts, but they are less broad and propose more specific outcomes. Theories guide propositions or relationship statements that are consistent with the model or framework from which they are derived, but a theory proposes an outcome that is more specific (e.g., theory of accelerating change, theory of the person as an adaptive system, or theory of goal attainment). When the nurse approaches people from the perspective of a certain nursing model and asks questions, processes information, and carries out activities in a certain way according to that model, a specific outcome is proposed based on the application of the theory of that model. Therefore the outcome is directly related to the model and theory that the nurse is using to guide the nursing care.

Rogers' theory of accelerating change, Roy's theory of the person as an adaptive system, and King's theory of goal attainment may be thought of as grand theories because of the abstract level of the theory in relation to the model from which they are derived. Grand theory is similar to what some have referred to descriptively as broad-range theory (Chinn & Kramer, 1995). When a theory is at the grand-theory level, many applications of that theory can be made in practice at the middle-range level by specifying such factors as the age of the patient, the situation, the health condition, the location, or the action of the nurse. This process of specifying the details of the theory makes it less abstract and less broad; therefore it applies to specific types of patients and makes specific propositions about the outcome of care.

Table 3-1 presents the knowledge structure with examples to illustrate these levels of nursing knowledge. The metaparadigm is the most abstract set of central concepts (i.e., person, environment, health, and nursing), and these concepts are defined by each conceptual model according to the philosophy of that model. Conceptual models (also called paradigms or frameworks) are the next less abstract set of concepts in the structure (e.g., King's systems framework). Grand theory is next as the level of abstraction descends (e.g., King's theory of goal attainment). Theory may be considered grand when it is nearly as abstract as the model itself and the usefulness of the model depends on the soundness of that theory. Grand theory is very useful in research and practice because more specific theory can be derived from it. Theory is the next less abstract level; it is more specific than grand theory but not as specific as middle-range theory (e.g., goal attainment in specific settings). Finally, as mentioned earlier, middle-range theory is the least abstract set of concepts and most specific to the details of nursing practice (e.g., goal attainment in adolescent, type II diabetic patients in the community).

The confusion in theory terminology in the nursing literature may, in addition to reflecting the various disciplines in which nurses receive higher education (as mentioned in Chapter 1), be explained by these different levels of abstraction of sets of concepts or by the different ways of naming theory (Alligood, 1994; Fawcett, 1989, 1995; Reynolds, 1971). Reynolds (1971) says that theory may be named for the person who authors it, for the outcome that it proposes, or for the shell of characteristics its content demarcates as an explanatory shell in isolation from other events in practice.

TABLE 3-1	Knowledge Structure Levels with Examples
Structure Level	**Example**
Metaparadigm	Person, environment, health, nursing
Conceptual models	King's systems framework
Grand theory	King's theory of goal attainment
Theory	Goal attainment in hospital settings
Middle-range theory	Goal attainment in adolescent diabetic patients in the community

Modified from Fawcett, J. (1989). *Analysis and evaluation of conceptual models of nursing* (2nd ed.). Philadelphia: F. A. Davis; Fawcett, J. (1993). *Analysis and evaluation of nursing theories*. Philadelphia: F. A. Davis.

In nursing there are examples of each of Reynolds' ways of naming theory (1971). In general, the author's name has been included in reference to the model as in King's systems framework; grand theory is named for the outcome it proposes as in the theory of goal attainment (King, 1981, 1995b); and the name of middle-range theory tends to include the explanatory shell of the characteristics of the content as in the theory of departmental power (Sieloff, 1991, 1995).

Each model provides a unique view for nursing practice that is specific to the model. Likewise, the theories derived from the model have propositions that are specific to the theory and are also consistent with the view of the model. Middle-range theory, which is the least abstract level, may be derived from the model, grand theory, or theory level. The relationship of nursing models and their theories is best illustrated by reviewing the nursing models individually along with the theories that have been derived from them.

Johnson's Behavioral System Model

When practicing nursing with the behavioral system model, the nurse views the person as a system of behaviors (Johnson, 1980). The actions and responses of the person comprise a system of interacting subsystems. Therefore assessment of the subsystems leads to an understanding of the whole behavior of the patient. Seven subsystems (see following box) are identified to understand the activities of the person.

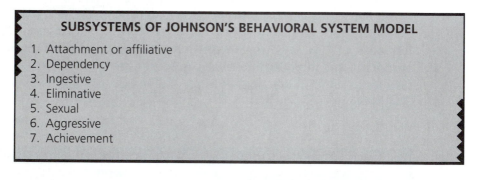

SUBSYSTEMS OF JOHNSON'S BEHAVIORAL SYSTEM MODEL

1. Attachment or affiliative
2. Dependency
3. Ingestive
4. Eliminative
5. Sexual
6. Aggressive
7. Achievement

Three theories from Johnson's behavioral system model are listed in the box at the top of p. 35. The theory of the person as a behavioral system is an implied grand theory of the model that has not been formalized. Two middle-range theories have been derived from the model: the theory of a restorative subsystem (Grubbs, 1974), proposed as an additional subsystem to the seven subsystem model developed by Johnson, and the theory of sustenal imperatives developed by Holaday, Turner-Henson, & Swan (in press) based on Grubbs' work (1974). Holaday illustrates the application of this model and her theory in nursing practice in Chapter 4.

THEORIES DERIVED FROM JOHNSON'S BEHAVIORAL SYSTEM MODEL

Theory of the person as a behavioral system
Theory of restorative subsystem (Grubbs, 1974)
Theory of sustenal imperatives (Holaday, Turner-Henson, & Swan, in press)

King's Systems Framework

Nurses practicing with King's systems framework think in terms of three interacting systems: a personal system, an interpersonal system, and a social system (King 1971, 1981, 1995a). Nursing practice in this framework is interactive, with the nurse viewing the patient as a personal system with interpersonal and social systems. King identifies each of the systems with a group of concepts, that, when considered together, specify the process of that system. The concepts of the three systems are presented in the following box.

SYSTEM CONCEPTS OF KING'S SYSTEMS FRAMEWORK

PERSONAL SYSTEM	INTERPERSONAL SYSTEM	SOCIAL SYSTEM
Perception	Interaction	Power
Self	Communication	Authority
Growth and development	Transaction	Status
Body image	Stress	Decision making
Time and space	Role	Role
		Organization

King (1981) developed the theory of goal attainment from her own systems framework. Her theory that perceptual congruence and transactions in the nurse/patient interaction lead to goal attainment as a nursing outcome has been used in different areas of nursing practice (Alligood, 1995; Hanna, 1995). Two other theories (see box below) were derived from King's system framework by Frey (1989) and Seiloff (1991, 1995). Frey and Norris present case applications in Chapter 5.

THEORIES DERIVED FROM KING'S SYSTEMS FRAMEWORK

Theory of goal attainment
Theory of social support and health (Frey, 1989)
Theory of departmental power (Sieloff, 1991, 1995)

Levine's Conservation Model

Nursing practice with the conservation model and principles focuses on conserving the patient's energy for health and healing (Levine 1967, 1991). The principles (see following box) constitute conservation for the whole person when considered together.

LEVINE'S CONSERVATION PRINCIPLES

1. Conservation of energy
2. Conservation of structural integrity
3. Conservation of personal integrity
4. Conservation of social integrity

Three theories have been derived from Levine's model (see box below). The first is a grand theory of conservation, which is implicit from the model and principles but has not yet been fully explicated. Two middle-range theories have been proposed by Levine: the theory of redundancy, which explains the fail-safe systems of the human body, and the theory of therapeutic intention. Of these two theories, the theory of therapeutic intention has been noted by Schaefer (1991) as very relevant to nursing practice because of its linkage to intervention. She has practiced with Levine's model, principles, and theories and written about their use in research, education, and practice. She illustrates the utilization of Levine's model and conservation principles in nursing practice with case applications in Chapter 6.

THEORIES DERIVED FROM LEVINE'S MODEL

Theory of conservation
Theory of therapeutic intention
Theory of redundancy

Neuman's Systems Model

When practicing nursing with the Neuman systems model (1972, 1982, 1989, 1995), the nurse thinks of the client in terms of a system of variables interacting with the environment while focusing on stressors as they relate to client health. The nurse views the client with a central core of five variables: physiological, psychological, sociocultural, developmental, and spiritual. The variables interact systematically with the lines of resistance, normal line of defense, and the flexible line of defense as the client system acts or responds in a wholistic manner with intrapersonal, interpersonal, and extrapersonal stressors.

Two theories (see following box) have been derived from the model: the theory of optimal client stability and the theory of prevention as intervention (Neuman, 1995). The theory of optimal client stability is very useful with multiple client changes. The theory of prevention as intervention is inherent in the systematic model since interventions are focused on increasing awareness of stress and stress reduction for a prevention outcome. Both theories are useful in practice since nursing action is linked to a nursing outcome for the client. These broad theories have numerous applications when age, health status, and nature of stressors are specified. Sohier demonstrates the application of Neuman's systems model in the nursing care of Debbie and homeless women in Chapter 7.

THEORIES DERIVED FROM NEUMAN'S SYSTEMS MODEL

Theory of optimal client stability
Theory of prevention as intervention

Orem's Conceptual Model

Nursing practice according to Orem's conceptual model (Orem, 1971, 1980, 1985, 1991, 1995) is a deliberate action of the nurse who views patients in terms of their self-care capacity. The concepts of Orem's model of nursing are presented in the following box.

CONCEPTS OF OREM'S MODEL

MAJOR CONCEPTS	PERIPHERAL CONCEPT
Self-care	Basic conditioning factors
Self-care agency	
Therapeutic self-care demand	
Self-care deficit	
Nursing agency	
Nursing system	

Orem has specified the relationships of her concepts in a set of theories: self-care, self-care deficit, and nursing system (see box at the top of p. 38). These three theories articulate to form an overall theory Orem calls self-care deficit theory (Orem, 1995, p. 170). The three theories form a system of complementary theories to guide nursing action. The theories specify self-care and therapeutic self-care demand in relation to self-care requisites, or patient variables, and nursing agency, which is the nurse variable. The conceptual model with the system of theories provides guidance specific to patient activity and nursing action whether the patient is capable of self-care or needs compensation of care. Berbiglia illustrates practice with Orem's theories in Chapter 8.

> ## OREM'S THEORIES
>
> Self-care deficit theory or general theory of nursing
>   Theory of self-care deficit or dependent-care deficit
>   Theory of self-care
>   Theory of nursing systems

Rogers' Science of Unitary Human Beings

When practice is based on the science of unitary human beings (Rogers, 1970, 1986, 1990, 1992), the systematic focus is the life process or pattern of the human being. The four concepts are openness, energy field, pattern, and pandimensionality. The three homeodynamic principles—helicy, resonancy, and integrality—describe the relationship of the main concepts.

Many theories have been derived from Rogers' science of unitary human beings. The conceptual system and its theories guide research, education, and practice (Alligood, 1990, 1991). The first four theories listed in the box below were derived by Rogers. The science of unitary human beings has also been used by others to generate theory as noted in the box. Besides testing the theories derived by the theorist, the researcher may also develop a theory from either the model or a grand theory already proposed (Fawcett, 1993). Bultemeier's theory of perception of dissonant pattern (1993) is an example of a middle-range theory derived from Rogers' theory of accelerating change and tested in women who reported experiencing premenstrual syndrome (PMS). Bultemeier illustrates the use of the science of unitary human beings in her nursing practice with women in Chapter 9.

> ## THEORIES DERIVED FROM ROGERS' SCIENCE OF UNITARY HUMAN BEINGS
>
> Theory of accelerating change
> Theory of paranormal phenomena
> Theory of rhythmical correlates of change
> Theory of aging
>
> Theory of health as expanding consciousness (Newman, 1995)
> Theory of human becoming (Parse, 1992)
> Theory of human field motion (Ference, 1986)
> Theory of power (Barrett, 1989)
> Theory of perceived dissonance (Bultemeier, 1993)

Roy's Adaptation Model

When nursing practice is based on the adaptation model, the focus is on the person as an adaptive system (Roy 1980, 1984; Roy & Roberts, 1981; Roy & Andrews, 1991). Adaptation is through cognator and regulator control processes, which lead to coping behavior in four modes: physiological mode, self-concept mode, role function mode, and interdependence mode.

Roy has developed a theory of the person as an adaptive system, and each of the four modes is also presented as a theory (see box below). In terms of their specificity to nursing practice, the theory of the person as an adaptive system is a grand theory and the theories of the four modes are middle-range theories specific to the modes of coping.

Phillips (1994) tested a middle-range theory from Roy's adaptation model and her theory of the person as an adaptive system. He formed a middle-range theory of adaptation of persons living with AIDS. His work is an example of how a middle-range theory derives from a grand theory and specifies an outcome (coping in the four modes) in a specific patient population (persons living with AIDS). Phillips illustrates the use of Roy's model and theories in nursing practice with Debbie and a case presentation from his practice with AIDS patients in Chapter 10.

THEORIES DERIVED FROM ROY'S ADAPTATION MODEL

Theory of the person as an adaptive system
Theory of the physiological mode
Theory of the self-concept mode
Theory of the interdependence mode
Theory of the role function mode

NURSING MODELS AND CRITICAL THINKING

As the nursing profession continues to develop, it has become quite clear that critical thinking and professional nursing practice are inextricably linked. When nursing theory guides the critical thinking of the decision-making process, it brings the knowing and doing of the nurse together in a nursing framework. Therefore theory utilization is essential to this phase of the development of the nursing profession since theory provides the basis for the nurse's knowing as well as a structure to guide nursing action (Mitchell, 1992; Sparacino, 1991).

Kuhn (1970) has said that it is the study of the models or paradigms of a scientific discipline that primarily prepares students for practice as members of that professional community. The paradigm (model or framework) plays a vital role in practice because without a framework all of the information that the professional encounters seems to be equally relevant. Therefore students studying to enter a professional discipline are introduced to the models or paradigms as an orientation to the approaches used in the practice of that discipline. Following an introduction and survey of the models, students are ready to choose the model or models they will use in their practice. It is in studying these models and practicing with them that students "learn their trade" (Kuhn, 1970, p. 43).

Critical thinking has been included in nursing curricula in the past, but it has moved to a position of prominence as a required criterion in the latest National League for Nursing Baccalaureate and Higher Degree Programs Accreditation Criteria (1992). This emphasis on critical thinking is not limited to nursing. Critical thinking has become a prevalent topic and research focus in higher education in the last decade. This is reflected in the formation of a National Council for Excellence in Critical Thinking Instruction. That council adopted the following working definition of critical thinking as presented by Paul and Nosich (1991):

> Critical thinking is the intellectually disciplined process of actively and skillfully conceptualizing, applying, analyzing, synthesizing, or evaluating information gathered from, or generated by, observation, experience, reflection, reasoning, or communication, as a guide to belief and action (p. 4).

The fact that nursing is a profession that is carried out for a certain purpose, according to the laws governing nursing practice in each state, makes it a purposeful activity. Further, the fact that nursing is an activity that answers a social mandate to determine an outcome from intelligible reasoning permits nursing to meet the criterion required for critical or higher order thinking.

"Elements of thought, macro-abilities, traits of mind or affective dimensions and intellectual standards" have been proposed as the domains of critical thinking (Paul and Nosich, 1991, pp. 2-3). Nursing models have been identified to guide the reasoning of critical thinking (Alligood, 1994; Field, 1987; Mayberry, 1991; Sorrentino, 1991). A comparison of the eight elements of thought in critical thinking and nursing thought with nursing models supports the premise as illustrated in Table 3-2.

As we move to the theory utilization phase of the theory era, the continuous development of the discipline of nursing becomes more evident. The process and content of nursing that have often been viewed separately are now folded together in a unique way in theory-based critical thinking. We move beyond the nursing process emphasis as we have known it, with its linear focus on what the nurse does in relation to the physiology and social science views of the patient, to a view of the whole person and a nursing approach to practice. Actually the processes— nursing process, research process, and theory development process—all

TABLE 3-2 Comparison of Critical Thinking and Nursing Thought

Elements of Thought in Critical Thinking	Nursing Thought
1. Purpose, goal, or end in view	Patient health
2. Question at issue or problem	Health at risk
3. Point of view/frame of reference	Whole persons
4. Empirical dimensions	Person, environment, health, and nursing
5. Conceptual dimensions	Derived from model
6. Assumptions	Derived from model
7. Implications	Derived from model
8. Inferences	Derived from model

beg the question: "Process of what?" Theory-guided practice based on a nursing model provides an answer to that question because the model specifies the content as well as the process of nursing practice and guides both the thought and the action. Therefore when viewed in the context of nursing practice, the processes become the tools of practice.

Mayberry (1991) calls for a merging of models, theories, and nursing practice and says, "Theories and models reveal the relationship of one part of nursing to another. They provide a systematic approach for thinking about nursing matters, for observing the nursing situation, and for interpreting what is seen in the practice setting" (p. 47). Levine (1995) has called for a demonstration of how theory illuminates care as it specifies a perspective of the person, nursing action, and an expected outcome. Utilization of theory in practice has been noted as its most important function (Stevens, 1984; as cited in Sorrentino, 1991). Similarly, Kerlinger (1979) has said "that the most important influence on practice is theory" (p. 296). Therefore theory-guided critical thinking is foundational to nursing practice (Mitchell, 1992).

SELECTING A MODEL FOR NURSING PRACTICE

The information presented so far forms a basis for selecting a model or theory for practice. But, besides knowledge of the models and their theories and understanding how they relate and how they form critical thinking structures to guide nursing practice, there is one additional factor to consider when selecting a model for nursing practice. There needs to be a "fit" between the values inherent in the model and one's personal values. Identification of one's personal values and the values within the model help the nurse to identify the model best suited to his/her practice. It is important to select a model or theory carefully to serve as a tool for the reasoning process of professional practice.

One may find writing a brief philosophy of nursing clarifies beliefs and values. This exercise can be done using the headings of person, environment, health, and nursing, for example. The process of thinking through and writing a philosophy forces one to consider what beliefs and values one truly holds. Once beliefs are clarified, a survey of the definitions of person, environment, health, and nursing in the various models and theories leads one to particular models or theories to be considered. Reviewing the assumptions of the model and comparing them with one's philosophy identifies linkage between the model and one's values and beliefs. This process may be undertaken by considering whether the concepts of the model are focused on similar aspects of the patient, aspects of nursing, or a view of health that one values.

This evaluation leads to the next step, which is to explore the particular models in depth. This process is a bit like "trying them on." One should consider the models that have been identified by making several applications in a selected area of nursing practice. By comparing two or three models on client focus, nursing action, and proposed outcome, one will find that a more in-depth understanding of the models emerges. Review the nursing literature written by authors who have used the models in their practice and research. Reviewing model applications in various areas highlights the flexibility of the model. Select a model and develop its use for your practice. As your practice with the model becomes more natural, tailor it to the special aspects of the art of nursing as you practice it. These guidelines (see box below) may be used to identify a model for theory-based nursing practice. The first step toward theory-based practice is the decision to do so (Mathwig, 1975). It takes commitment to develop a base of understanding (Marriner-Tomey, 1994).

GUIDELINES FOR SELECTING A MODEL FOR NURSING PRACTICE

1. Consider values and beliefs truly held in nursing.
2. Write a philosophy of beliefs on person, environment, health, and nursing.
3. Survey definitions of person, environment, health, and nursing in the nursing models.
4. Select two or three models that link best with your values.
5. Review the assumptions of the models you have selected.
6. Make applications of those models in a selected area of nursing practice (try them out).
7. Compare the models on client focus, nursing action, and client outcome.
8. Review the nursing literature written by persons who have used the models in nursing practice and research.
9. Select a model and develop its use in your practice.

References

Alligood, M. R. (1990). Nursing care of the elderly: Futuristic projections. In E. A. M. Barrett (Ed.), *Visions of Rogers' science-based nursing* (pp. 129-141). New York: National League for Nursing.

Alligood, M. R. (1991). Testing Rogers' theory of accelerating change: The relationships among creativity, actualization, and empathy in persons 18-92 years of age. *Western Journal of Nursing Research, 13*(1), 84-96.

Alligood, M. R. (1994). Evolution of nursing theory development. In A. Marriner-Tomey (Ed.), *Nursing theorists and their work* (3rd ed., pp. 58-69). St. Louis: Mosby.

Alligood, M. R. (1995). Theory of goal attainment: Application to adult orthopedic nursing. In M. Frey & C. Sieloff (Eds.), *Advancing King's systems framework and theory of nursing* (pp. 209-222). Thousand Oaks, CA: Sage Publications.

Barrett, E. A. M. (1989). A theory of power for nursing practice: Derivation from Rogers' paradigm. In J. P. Riehl-Sisca (Ed.), *Conceptual models for nursing practice* (3rd ed., pp. 207-217). Norwalk, CT: Appleton & Lange.

Bultemeier, K. I. (1993). *Photographic inquiry of the phenomenon premenstrual syndrome within a Rogerian-derived theory of perceived dissonance.* Unpublished doctoral dissertation, University of Tennessee, Knoxville, TN.

Carper, B. (1978). Fundamental patterns of knowing. *Advances in Nursing Science, 1*(1), 13-23.

Chinn, P., & Kramer, M. (1995). *Theory and nursing: A systematic approach* (3rd ed.). St. Louis: Mosby.

Fawcett, J. (1989). *Analysis and evaluation of conceptual models of nursing* (2nd ed.). Philadelphia: F. A. Davis.

Fawcett, J. (1993). *Analysis and evaluation of nursing theories.* Philadelphia: F. A. Davis.

Fawcett, J. (1995). *Analysis and evaluation of conceptual models of nursing* (3rd ed.). Philadelphia: F. A. Davis.

Ference, H. (1986). The relationship of time experience, creativity traits, differentiation, and human field motion. In V. M. Malinski (Ed.), *Explorations on Martha Rogers' science of unitary human beings* (pp. 95-106). Norwalk, CT: Appleton-Century-Crofts.

Field, P. A. (1987). The impact of nursing theory on the clinical decision making process. *Journal of Advanced Nursing, 12,* 563-571.

Frey, M. A. (1989). Social support and health: A theoretical formulation derived from King's conceptual framework. *Nursing Science Quarterly, 2,* 138-148.

Grubbs, J. (1974). An interpretation of the Johnson behavioral system model. In J. P. Riehl & C. Roy (Eds.), *Conceptual models for nursing practice* (pp. 160-197). Norwalk, CT: Appleton-Century-Crofts.

Hanna, K. M. (1995). Use of King's theory of goal attainment to promote adolescents' health behavior. In M. A. Frey & C. L. Sieloff (Eds.), *Advancing King's systems framework and theory of nursing* (pp. 239-250). Thousand Oaks, CA: Sage Publications.

Holaday, B. (1974). Achievement behavior in chronically ill children. *Nursing Research, 23,* 25-30.

Holaday, B., Turner-Henson, A., & Swan, J. (in press). Explaining activities of chronically ill children: An analysis using the Johnson behavioral system model. In P. Hinton-Walker & B. Neuman (Eds.), *Blueprint for use of nursing models.* New York: National League for Nursing.

Johnson, D. E. (1980). The behavioral system model for nursing. In J. P. Riehl & C. Roy (Eds.), *Conceptual models for nursing practice* (pp. 207-216). Norwalk, CT: Appleton-Century-Crofts.

Kerlinger, F. N. (1979). *Behavioral research: A conceptual approach.* New York: Holt Rinehart & Winston.

King, I. (1971). *Toward a theory for nursing: General concepts of human behavior.* New York: John Wiley & Sons.

King, I. (1981). *A theory for nursing: Systems, concepts, process.* New York: John Wiley & Sons.

King, I. (1995a). A systems framework for nursing. In M. Frey & C. Sieloff (Eds.), *Advancing King's systems framework and theory of nursing* (pp. 14-22). Thousand Oaks, CA: Sage Publications.

King, I. (1995b). The theory of goal attainment. In M. Frey & C. Sieloff (Eds.), *Advancing King's systems framework and theory of nursing* (pp. 23-32). Thousand Oaks, CA: Sage Publications.

Kuhn, T. S. (1970). *The structure of scientific revolutions* (2nd ed.). Chicago: University of Chicago Press.

Levine, M. E. (1967). The four conservation principles of nursing. *Nursing Forum, 6,* 45-59.

Levine, M. (1988). *The nursing theorist: Portraits of excellence* [video]. Oakland, CA: Studio III.

Levine, M. E. (1991). The conservation principles: A model for health. In K. M. Schaefer & J. A. B. Pond (Eds.), *Levine's conservation model: A framework for nursing practice* (pp. 1-11). Philadelphia: F. A. Davis.

Levine, M. E. (1995). The rhetoric of nursing theory. *IMAGE: Journal of Nursing Scholarship, 27*(1), 11-14.

Marriner-Tomey, A. (1994). Preface. In A. Marriner-Tomey (Ed.), *Nursing theorists and their work* (3rd ed., pp. xi-xii). St. Louis: Mosby.

Mathwig, G. (1975). Translation of nursing science theory to nursing education. In S. Ketefian, (Ed.), *Translation of theory into nursing practice and education.* Proceedings of the Seventh Annual Clinical Sessions, Continuing Education in Nursing Division of School of Education, Health, Nursing, and Arts Professions, New York University.

Mayberry, A. (1991). Merging nursing theories, models, and nursing practice: More than an administrative challenge. *Nursing Administration Quarterly, 15*(3), 44-53.

Mitchell, G. (1992). Specifying the knowledge base of theory in practice. *Nursing Science Quarterly, 5*(1), 6-7.

National League for Nursing. (1992). *Criteria and guidelines for the evaluation of baccalaureate and higher degree programs in nursing* (7th ed). New York: Author.

Neuman, B. & Young, R. (1972). A model for teaching total person approach to patient problems. *Nursing Research, 21,* 264-269.

Neuman, B. (1982). *The Neuman systems model.* Norwalk, CT: Appleton-Century-Crofts.

Neuman, B. (1989). *The Neuman systems model* (2nd ed.). Norwalk, CT: Appleton & Lange.

Neuman, B. (1995). *The Neuman systems model* (3rd ed.). Norwalk, CT: Appleton & Lange.

Newman, M. (1995). *Health as expanding consciousness.* New York: Nursing League for Nursing.

Orem, D. E. (1971). *Nursing: Concepts of practice.* New York: McGraw-Hill.

Orem, D. E. (1980). *Nursing: Concepts of practice* (2nd ed.). New York: McGraw-Hill.

Orem, D. E. (1985). *Nursing: Concepts of practice* (3rd ed.). New York: McGraw-Hill.

Orem, D. E. (1991). *Nursing: Concepts of practice* (4th ed.). St. Louis: Mosby.

Orem, D. E. (1995). *Nursing: Concepts of practice* (5th ed.). St. Louis: Mosby.

Parse, R. (1992). Human becoming: Parse's theory of nursing. *Nursing Science Quarterly, 5,* 35-42.

Paul, R. W., & Nosich, G. M. (1991). *Proposal for the national assessment of higher-order thinking* (revised version). The United States Department of Education Office of Educational Research and Improvement, National Center for Education Statistics.

Phillips, K. D. (1994). *Testing biobehavioral adaptation in person living with AIDS using Roy's theory of the person as an adaptive system.* Unpublished doctoral dissertation, University of Tennessee, Knoxville, TN.

Reynolds, P. (1971). *A primer in theory construction.* Indianapolis: Bobbs-Merril.

Rogers, M. E. (1970). *An introduction to the theoretical basis of nursing.* Philadelphia: F. A. Davis.

Rogers, M. E. (1986). Science of unitary human beings. In V. M. Malinski (Ed.), *Explorations on Martha Rogers' science of unitary human beings* (pp. 3-8). Norwalk, CT: Appleton & Lange.

Rogers, M. E. (1990). Nursing: Science of unitary, irreducible, human beings: Update 1990. In E. A. M. Barrett (Ed.), *Visions of Rogers' science-based nursing* (pp. 5-11). New York: National League for Nursing.

Rogers, M. E. (1992). Nursing science and the space age. *Nursing Science Quarterly, 5,* 27-34.

Roy, C. (1980). The Roy adaptation model. In J. P. Riehl & C. Roy (Eds.), *Conceptual models for nursing practice* (2nd ed., pp. 179-188). Norwalk, CT: Appleton-Century-Crofts.

Roy, C. (1984). *Introduction to nursing: An adaptation model* (2nd ed.). Englewood Cliffs, NJ: Prentice-Hall.

Roy, C., & Andrews, H. (1991). *The Roy adaptation model: The definitive statement.* Norwalk, CT: Appleton & Lange.

Roy, C., & Roberts, S. L. (1981). *Theory construction in nursing: An adaptation model.* Englewood Cliffs, NJ: Prentice-Hall.

Schaefer, K. (1991). Levine's conservation principles and research. In K. M. Schaefer & J. A. B. Pond (Eds.), *Levine's conservation model: A framework for nursing practice* (pp. 45-59). Philadelphia: F. A. Davis.

Sieloff, C. (1991). *Imogene King: A conceptual framework for nursing.* Thousand Oaks, CA: Sage Publications.

Sieloff, C. (1995). Development of a theory of departmental power. In M. Frey & C. Sieloff (Eds.), *Advancing King's systems framework and theory of nursing* (pp. 46-65). Thousand Oaks, CA: Sage Publications.

Sorrentino, E. A. (1991). Making theories work for you. *Nursing Administration Quarterly, 15*(3), 54-59.

Sparacino, P. (1991). The reciprocal relationship between practice and theory. *Clinical Nurse Specialist, 5*(3), 138.

Application

The application of models and theories in nursing practice illustrates their utility.

Each theoretical model provides a unique perspective to guide the nursing care of Debbie:

- A system of behaviors when Johnson is applied
- A framework of interacting systems when King is applied
- A set of conservation principles when Levine is applied
- A system response to stressors when Neuman is applied
- A set of theories for self-care when Orem is applied
- A human/environmental field pattern when Rogers is applied
- A system of adaptive modes when Roy is applied

Each theoretical model is further illustrated by utilization and application with a selected case of the author's choice.

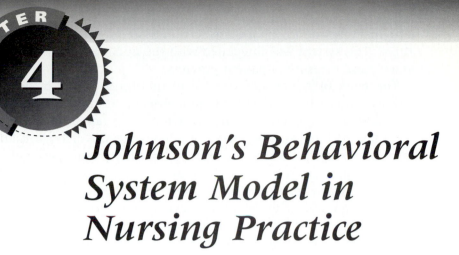

Johnson's Behavioral System Model in Nursing Practice

Bonnie Holaday

Nursing is *"an external regulatory force that acts to preserve the organization and integration of the patient's behavior at an optimal level under those conditions in which the behavior constitutes a threat to physical or social health or in which illness is found."* The goal of nursing is to *"restore, maintain or attain behavioral integrity, system stability, adjustment and adaptation, efficient and effective functioning of the system." (Johnson, 1980).*

HISTORY AND BACKGROUND

The Johnson's behavioral system model (JBSM) was conceived and developed by Dorothy Johnson while she was a professor of nursing at the University of California, Los Angeles. The process of developing this model began in the late 1950s as she examined the explicit goal of action of patient welfare that was unique to nursing. The task was to clarify nursing's social mission from the perspective of a theoretically sound view of the client. The conceptual model that resulted was presented at Vanderbilt University in 1968 (Johnson, 1968). Since that time there have been other noteworthy presentations of the model (Auger, 1976; Derdiarian, 1990, 1993; Dee, 1990; Grubbs, 1974; Johnson, 1980, 1990).

The JBSM has provided useful guidelines for nursing practice. When used in conjunction with the nursing process, it has provided a useful conceptual map to plan patient care. Auger and Dee (1983) provided evidence supporting the efficacy of the JBSM as a tool for evaluating nursing interventions. These authors developed the UCLA Neuropsychiatric Institute and Hospital Classification System, which is based on the JBSM. This system was integrated with the nursing process and is used as a clinical measure of patient progress.

The work of Auger and Dee led to the development of behavioral indices, with each subsystem operationalized in terms of critical adaptive and maladaptive behaviors. The behaviors were ranked into categories according to their assumed level of adaptiveness. Nurse clinicians can rate each behavior for compliance with an activity rating scale of 1 to 4. This scale provided a basis for allocating nursing resources at the UCLA Neuropsychiatric Institute (Dee & Randell, 1989).

Derdiarian used the JBSM to develop the Derdiarian Behavioral System model (DBSM) instrument (Derdiarian, 1983, 1988; Derdiarian & Forsythe, 1983). The DBSM's 22-category interview generated data pertaining to the major changes in the behavioral systems as a result of illness as well as the positive or negative effects of these changes. Specifically, two types of subjective data were generated. This included the "set"-related variables or the variables that potentially predict or influence the patient's usual behavior and the behavior resulting from illness. Overall, her research findings suggested that using the DBSM instrument in the nursing process improved the focus, comprehensiveness, and quality of nursing assessment, diagnoses, interventions and evaluation of outcomes of adult patients with cancer, AIDS, and myocardial infarction.

Other articles have also documented the utility of the JBSM for nursing practice. Holaday (1980) used the model to assess health status and to develop nursing interventions for children undergoing surgical procedures. Rawls (1980) used the model to develop a nursing care plan for an adult amputee with a body image problem. Majeslty, Brester, and Nishio (1978) used the JBSM to develop an instrument to measure patient indicators of nursing care, and Glennin (1980) also developed standards for nursing practice from Johnson's conceptual model. Riegel (1989) operationalized the JBSM to examine social support and adjustment to coronary heart disease.

Holaday's work demonstrated that subsystem disorders can be identified, validated the notion of behavioral subsystems and their utility and usefulness in nursing practice, broadened the understanding of the role of "set," and most recently examined the relationship between sustenal imperatives and action (Holaday 1974, 1981, 1982, 1987; Holaday, Turner-Henson, & Swan, in press). Derdiarian's research demonstrated the factor-isolating and categorizing potential of the JBSM, validated the notion of behavioral subsystems, and provided empirical descriptions of central concepts in the theory (Derdiarian, 1983, 1988, 1990; Derdiarian & Forsythe, 1983). Meleis (1991) described the body of research related to nursing practice that the JBSM has generated and noted that it has provided "significant developments in the conceptualization of the nursing client" (p. 269).

OVERVIEW OF JOHNSON'S BEHAVIORAL SYSTEM MODEL

Johnson's model for nursing presents a view of the client as a living open system. The client is seen as a collection of behavioral subsystems that interrelate to form a behavioral system. Therefore the behavior is the system, not the individual. This system of behavior is characterized by repetitive, regular, predictable, and goal-directed behaviors that always strive toward balance (Johnson, 1968).

Johnson (1968) proposed that the nursing client is a behavioral system with behaviors of interest to nursing organized into seven subsystems of behavior: achievement, affiliative, aggressive, dependence, eliminative, ingestive, sexual. Nurses (Grubbs, 1974; Auger, 1976; Derdiarian, 1990; Holaday, 1980) using the model believed an additional area of behavior needed to be addressed and added an eighth subsystem (restorative). Each subsystem has its own structure and function. The structure of each is comprised of a goal based on a universal drive, set, choice, and action. Each of these four factors contributes to the observable activity of a person.

The goal of a subsystem is defined as "the ultimate consequence of behaviors in it" (Grubbs, 1974, p. 226). The basis for the goal is a universal drive whose existence is supported by existing theory or research. The goal of each subsystem is the same for all people when stated in general terms; however, there are variations among individuals based on the value placed on the goal and drive strength.

The second structural component is set, which is a tendency to act in a certain way in a given situation. Once developed, sets are relatively stable. Set formation is influenced by such societal norms and variables as culture, family, values, perception, and cognitive abilities. Set can be divided into two types: preparatory set and perseverative set. Preparatory set describes what one focuses on in a situation. The perseverative set, which implies persistence, refers to the habits one maintains. The flexibility or rigidity of the set varies with each person. Set plays a major role in determining the choices a person makes and actions eventually taken.

Choice refers to the alternate behaviors the person considers for use in any given situation. A person's range of options may be broad or narrow and are influenced by such variables as age, sex, culture, and socioeconomic status.

The action is the observable behavior of the person. The actual behavior is restricted by the person's size and abilities. Here the concern is the efficiency and effectiveness of the behavior in goal attainment.

Each of the subsystems also has a function that is analogous to the physiology of biological systems (e.g., the urological system has both structural and functional components). The goal of the subsystem is a part of the structure and it is not entirely separate from its function.

In order for the eight subsystems to develop and maintain stability, each must have a constant supply of "functional requirements" or sustenal imperatives (Johnson, 1980, p. 212). The environment must supply the functional requirements/sustenal imperatives of protection from unwanted, disturbing stimuli; nurturance through giving input from the environment (e.g., food, caring, conditions that support growth and development), encouragement; and stimulation by experiences, events, and behavior that would "enhance growth and prevent stagnation" (Johnson, 1980, p. 212).

The subsystems maintain behavioral system balance as long as both the internal and external environments are orderly, organized, and predictable and each of the subsystems' goals are met. Behavioral system imbalance arises when there is a disturbance in structure, function, or functional regimen. The JBSM differentiates four diagnostic classifications to delineate these disturbances: insufficiency, discrepancy, incompatibility, and dominance.

Nursing has the goal of maintaining, restoring, or attaining a balance or a stability in the behavioral system or the system as a whole. Nursing acts as an "external regulatory force" to modify or change the structure or to provide ways in which subsystems fulfill the structure's functional requirement (Johnson, 1980, p. 214). Interventions directed toward restoring behavioral system balance would be directed toward repairing damaged structural units, with the nurse temporarily imposing regulatory and control measures or helping the client to develop or enhance their supplies of essential functional requirements.

CRITICAL THINKING IN NURSING PRACTICE WITH JOHNSON'S MODEL

Making wise choices about nursing care requires the ability to think critically—that is, to analyze the available information, make inferences, draw logical conclusions, and critically evaluate all relevant elements as well as the possible consequences of each nursing decision. From a constructivist perspective, when individuals are presented with complex information, they use their own existing knowledge and previous experience to help them make sense of the material. In particular, they make inferences, elaborate on the information by adding details, and generate relationships between and among the new information and the information already in memory. In short, they think critically about the new and old information (Pressley, 1992; Wittrock, 1990). The JBSM provides a useful framework for organizing information so that one can arrange information in a way that permits problem solving and care planning (Table 4-1).

The focus of the assessment process is to obtain knowledge regarding the client through interviews and observations of the patient and family. The purpose is to evaluate the present behavior in terms of past patterns to determine the impact of the present illness or perceived health threat and/or hospitalization on behavioral patterns and to establish the maximum possible level of health toward which an individual can strive. The behavioral systems analysis approach provides a comprehensive framework in which various types of data can be organized into a cohesive structure.

The assessment gathers specific knowledge regarding the structure and function of the eight subsystems (behavioral assessment) and those general and specific factors that supply the subsystems' functional requirements/sustenal imperatives (environmental assessment). Interview questions in both areas need to be theory based. For example, Piagetian theory can be used to develop questions to assess the child's ability to express knowledge about illness—eliminative subsystem (Holaday, 1980).

Once the interview has been completed, it is necessary to analyze the data (diagnostic analysis, Table 4-1) to identify those patterns of behavior that are adaptive and functional for the client and those that are maladaptive and indicate behavioral systems imbalance. One component of the analysis determines if there is congruency among all structural units. Congruency will be evidenced by stable, patterned behavior, whereas discrepancy among the various components will be evidenced by unstable and disorganized behavior. The second component examines how the functional requirements/sustenal imperatives may be influencing subsystem behavior. For example, what effect is family interaction style having on the client's affiliative subsystem? The latter analysis is critical because it plays an important role in determining how the nurse needs to function as an "external regulator."

The nursing diagnosis is a summary of the results for the analysis and describes the current level of behavioral system function. It serves as a guide for intervention planning by the nursing team. The overall objective of the nursing intervention is to establish regularities in the client's behavior so that the goal of each subsystem is met. The focus of the intervention will be on either a structural part of the subsystem or the supply of sustenal imperatives/functional requirements.

Identification of goals is essential to the evaluation of client outcomes

TABLE 4-1 The Johnson Model and the Nursing Process

Framework Elements	Nursing Thought
BEHAVIORAL ASSESSMENT	
Eight subsystems 　Achievement 　Affiliative 　Aggressive/protective 　Dependency 　Eliminative 　Ingestive 　Restorative 　Sexual	Do I understand the patient's perceptions? How complete are my data collections? Could I have missed something? How do I know I have the facts right? What data might need verifying? How do these data compare with previously collected data? How do my client's data compare with accepted standards/behaviors for someone of this age, culture, and disease process? What general and specific factors supply the functional requirements for the subsystems?
ENVIRONMENTAL ASSESSMENT	
Internal 　Biological 　Pathological 　Psychological 　Developmental 　Level of wellness External 　Cultural 　Ecological 　Familial 　Sociological	
DIAGNOSTIC ANALYSIS	
Behavior subsystem (e.g., achievement) Structural unit 　Goal, set, choice, action	What subsystem(s) is involved? What structural unit(s) is involved? Is behavior succeeding or failing to achieve the goal? Is there a clear relationship between the stated goal of the person, set, and chosen behavior? Does the set of the person result in misperception of the information? Are the choices appropriate? Is the sequence of action orderly and purposeful?
Sustenal imperatives 　Variables from the environment 　　(e.g., familial)	Which of the sustenal imperatives are causing or influencing the behavior(s)? What regulating and control mechanisms are present? What is the quality and quantity of sustenal imperatives?

TABLE 4-1 The Johnson Model and the Nursing Process—cont'd	
Framework Elements	**Nursing Thought**
DIAGNOSTIC ANALYSIS—cont'd	

Diagnostic label
  Insufficiency
  Discrepancy
  Incompatibility
  Dominance
	Questions to guide determination of diagnosis:
	What is the meaning of _____?
	What are the implications of _____?
	What do we already know about _____?
	How does _____ affect _____?
	Explain why _____?
	Explain how _____?
	Why is _____ important?
	What do you think causes _____? Why?
	What are the relationships between _____ and _____?

PLANNING AND INTERVENTION	
Mutual goal setting Identify focus of intervention Identify mode of intervention Identify technique	Questions to guide development of intervention: What would happen if _____? What are some possible interventions for the diagnosis of _____? What are possible unintended consequences of the intervention?
EVALUATION	
Establish long-term goals Establish short-term goals Develop behavioral objectives to measure progress toward goals	Are goals socially, culturally, and biologically appropriate? Are the goals reasonable? Are the goals client centered? Are the objectives measurable and theory based?

and for professional nursing care. To evaluate, the nurse must first predict expected client outcomes. This helps to ensure a purposeful, predictable course of client responses. To evaluate effectively, the nurse sets both long-term and short-term goals and behavioral objectives that will indicate that progress is being made toward achieving these goals.

ASE HISTORY OF DEBBIE

Debbie is a 29-year-old woman who was recently admitted to the oncology nursing unit for evaluation after sensing pelvic "fullness" and noticing a watery, foul-smelling vaginal discharge. A Papanicolaou smear revealed a class V cervical cancer. She was found to have a stage II squamous cell carcinoma of the cervix and underwent a radical hysterectomy with bilateral salpingooophorectomy.

Her past health history revealed that physical examinations had been infrequent. She also reported that she had not performed breast self-examination. She is 5 feet 4 inches tall and weighs 89 pounds. Her usual weight is about 110 pounds. She has smoked approximately two packs of cigarettes a day for the past 16 years. She is gravida 2, para 2. Her first pregnancy was at age 16, and her second was at age 18. Since that time she has taken oral contraceptives on a regular basis.

Debbie completed the eighth grade. She is married and lives with her husband and two children in her mother's home, which she describes as less than sanitary. Her husband is unemployed. She describes him as emotionally distant and abusive at times.

She has done well following surgery except for being unable to completely empty her urinary bladder. She is having continued postoperative pain and nausea. It will be necessary for her to perform intermittent self-catheterization at home. Her medications are (1) an antibiotic, (2) an analgesic as needed for pain, and (3) an antiemetic as needed for nausea. In addition, she will be receiving radiation therapy on an outpatient basis.

Debbie is extremely tearful. She expresses great concern over her future and the future of her two children. She believes that this illness is a punishment for her past life.

NURSING CARE OF DEBBIE WITH JOHNSON'S MODEL
Behavioral Assessment

The relevant behavioral assessment data are the following. *Achievement:* Debbie has an eighth grade education, feels a loss of control of her future and that of her children, and has a loss of ability to achieve the developmental outcomes of young adulthood. *Affiliative:* Debbie is married but describes her husband as emotionally distant and abusive at times; there may be a possible change in relationship. *Aggressive/Protective:* There may be a possible impairment of emotional endurance. Debbie is not protective of herself (smoked, sought healthcare infrequently, did not perform breast self-examination). With the loss of her health, she is protective of her children but her husband is unemployed (who will provide for family?). *Dependency:* Because she lives with her mother, there is a potential decrease in self-sufficiency. *Ingestive:* Debbie has experienced weight loss and nausea. *Eliminative:* Debbie is unable to empty her bladder. She is tearful, expressing concern about the future. *Sexual:* Because Debbie has had a hysterectomy, there may be a change in her sexual relationship with her husband and she may have concerns about her feminine identity. *Restorative:* Debbie is experiencing fatigue, pain, and possible sleep disturbance.

Diagnosis and intervention. The JBSM provides a perspective for nursing practice by viewing Debbie as a biopsychosocial being represented in a behavioral system. The subjective and objective data indicate a problem in the achievement subsystem. *Objective data:* Debbie has a class V cervical cancer-stage II squamous cell carcinoma of the cervix with an uncertain prognosis at this time. *Subjective data:* The patient is tearful and expressing concern about her ability to fulfill personal and family needs and responsibilities.

Environmental Assessment

The environmental assessment examines the sources of sustenal imperatives (functional requirements) to determine if they are providing the functional requirements needed to maintain behavioral system balance. If these are present (or have been present in sufficient quantity and quality over time), then the subsystems, and subsequently the entire system, operate at the same level of efficiency and effectiveness and are able to maintain overall balance and stability. If they are not present, the nurse will act as an external regulatory force to provide protection, stimulation, or nurturance; change structural units; or impose external regulatory mechanisms. The critical component of the environmental assessment is to identify the factors that are causing or influencing behavioral system problems.

The environmental assessment identifies several key factors. From a developmental perspective, Debbie is relatively young and thus many of the developmental tasks of young adulthood such as raising her children and establishing an occupation or career and other future plans could be impaired. The diagnosis of cancer raises questions about her physical ability to achieve personal goals, and the pain, fatigue, and anxiety may impair her mental ability to achieve personal goals. During the first 3 months following diagnosis, Debbie needs to address issues related to the diagnosis, including dying, the future, and the meaning life has had (Weisman, 1979). During this same time, Debbie will be presented with a treatment plan and will be simultaneously learning to cope with recovery from surgery and side effects of cancer therapy and planning for the future. The significance of this initial period cannot be overemphasized as Debbie attempts to regain control over herself and the environment.

Diagnosis and intervention. In examining Debbie's perseveratory set, one would note that Debbie's perception of herself as an independent agent generally capable of accomplishing her tasks and goals has been substantially altered. In terms of the preparatory set, her situational context is also substantially altered. She is most likely unclear about her choices. The diagnosis is insufficiency in the achievement subsystem. In terms of intervention, the nurse may function to protect Debbie from noxious stimuli because she is not able to cope with all situations at present. The nurse can provide nurturance in terms of providing counseling and help with goal setting. Stimulation in terms of teaching new self-care behaviors can also help. The biological disease process is unique for each person, and the psychosocial response to mastering the situation will be equally unique. Thus frequent reassessment and revision of the care plan will be needed.

Most patients faced with a diagnosis of cancer experience a life crisis. Although death is often the first fear, the potential for other stressors exists. Surgery, adjuvant therapy (radiation), the possible spread of malignancy, and an uncertain prognosis are all stressors. Surgery may lead to an altered body image with accompanying feelings of a loss of femininity. It is reasonable to assume that Debbie is experiencing some sexual concerns, and there should be a thorough assessment of the sexual subsystem since objective data indicate the potential for behavioral system imbalance.

The objective data identify that Debbie had a radical hysterectomy, which means the vaginal canal has been shortened. Sexual intercourse may be uncomfortable since the trigone of the bladder and sigmoid colon may be closely associated with the new vaginal apex. Debbie will receive radiation therapy. Side effects from this therapy may include fatigue, nausea and vomiting, impaired vaginal membrane integrity, bleeding, sexual dysfunction, and infection. The subjective data indicate that Debbie's husband is emotionally distant and abusive at times and that Debbie is tearful and worried about the future. When the perseveratory set is examined, it is clear that the current physiological functioning of the sex organs has been disrupted. Past socialization and experience in sex role behaviors may no longer seem applicable to Debbie. Within the context of the present situation (preparatory set), Debbie is most likely unclear where to direct her attention. The selection of a sexual behavior (choice) to meet goals is unclear.

The diagnosis of insufficiency could be made since the subsystem is not functioning to its fullest capacity. If Debbie takes actions that do not meet the intended goal of the subsystem, then a diagnosis of discrepancy could also be made.

Evaluation

Debbie has a knowledge deficit related to radiation therapy and needs nurturance in terms of education to help her understand and cope with the situation. A careful assessment needs to be conducted to determine

Debbie's understanding of the purpose and goal of treatment. Debbie needs to be taught preventive health practices that decrease the risk of impaired vaginal membrane integrity and comfort measures such as sitz baths and compresses to the perineum. Alternative methods of sexual intercourse can be discussed since sexual intercourse during treatment is encouraged to prevent adhesions and to prevent shortening of the vagina. Counseling with Debbie and her husband can help them create their own special intimacy, sense of affection, and physical gratification. The nurse's goal of helping to restore the patient's sexual function is tied in closely with goals of restoring or maintaining self-image and self-esteem.

ASE HISTORY OF MARK

Mark Fritz is a 12-year-old boy with myleomeningocele and neurogenic bladder. He was also diagnosed with diabetes at 9 years of age. He is admitted for a bladder augmentation and placement of an artificial sphincter. Mark has been hospitalized many times for surgical procedures (shunt revisions and orthopedic procedures). His mother and father are both present during the interview although Mrs. Fritz does most of the talking. Mark is also interviewed alone. Mark's brothers, Bill (17 years) and David (15 years), will visit him in the evenings but are not present during the admission interview.

NURSING CARE OF MARK WITH JOHNSON'S MODEL
Behavioral Assessment

Achievement. Mark looked at me and interacted with a great little smile when he described his school and how it is different. He describes it as a "handicap school." He likes it because there are only "16 kids and two teachers and I get lots of help." He is also proud of what he can do on the computer. Mark attributes his success to the presence or absence of ability and attributes little to motivational factors. He enjoyed the Piagetian testing, which place him in the concrete operations period. Both the nursing staff and his mother note that he requires verbal prompts to perform self-care activities. His mother notes that he has missed a lot of school during the past 2 years and that is why she and her husband removed Mark from regular public school and placed him in a special education school. The classes are ungraded, but his mother said he has made great progress at this school and now reads at a sixth grade level and has math skills at a fifth grade level. Mark is worried about "getting behind" while he is in the hospital. Mark has no idea what he wants to be when he grows up. He has not been to camp nor has he ever spent the night at another child's home. Mark has never been home alone; parent or sibling is always present.

Affiliative. Mark seems emotionally more attached to his mother than his father. He likes and admires his older brothers and wishes he "could ride dirt bikes with them." He spends a lot of time at home with his mother and alone watching TV or "messing around on the computer." He watches football games and other sports on TV with his father on the weekends. Mark cannot name a friend at his school or in his neighborhood. His mother states he likes to be "with other kids" and likes when his brothers' friends are at the house. She also could not name a child who was a friend. The nursing staff and his mother describe Mark as shy and my observation in the playroom confirms this. He is more talkative when his mother is absent. When she is present, Mark lets his mother answer questions or asks her to do so.

Aggressive/protective. His mother and the nursing staff describe him as passive and more likely to sulk than get angry. When I asked what he would do if someone took something of his or hit him, Mark said he "wouldn't like it."

Dependency. Mark refused to answer my questions about self-care. The nursing staff state they saw little evidence of self-care activity during previous admissions. He lets the nursing staff or his mother do them (maintain blood sugar, give insulin, select menu, perform bowel and bladder care). Mark's mother states that he has become more dependent on her during the past year. He asks for help to dress in addition to the above. The staff has noted more independent behavior when the mother and grandmother are absent. There was a tremendous difference between the way he acted with me when the mother and grandmother were not present (adult/child to adult/parent with me and child/parent with mother and grandmother).

Ingestive. Mark states "I like to eat." His mother also describes Mark as "loving food" and "eating too much." The switch to the "diabetic diet has been difficult for him." The family eats meals together. Postoperatively he usually has nausea and vomiting and fluid and food intake are poor. Mark is very observant of what goes on around him. He likes to "have tests and things explained" to him when he is in the hospital.

Eliminative. Mark has minimal bowel and bladder control. He has frequent problems with dribbling of urine. Mark himself admits this bothers him. His mother suspects he does not perform intermittent self-catheterization regularly at school because he is embarrassed about sexual changes and the fact that he must wear sanitary protection pads. As for his communication pattern, Mark tucks his head to his chest and mumbles when he is talking about his feelings or parents. Sometimes he simply refuses to answer or looks away. I suspect the game of mumbling and shyness is a means of coping with an overtalkative and overprotective mother and grandmother.

Restorative. Mark sleeps 8 hours a night but less in the hospital "because they wake you up all the time." He usually gets up around 7 AM on school days and 8:30 AM on the weekends. He has a somewhat restricted repertoire of interests and activities. He watches a lot of television and rented videos and plays computer games. He participates in no groups, clubs, or regular physical activity. He enjoys family weekend trips to the lake and dune buggy and boat rides.

Sexual. Mark looked away when I asked about changes in his body and "becoming a man." He did not answer my questions. He said he did not like "wearing special pants." When asked who he was most like in his family, he said his mother. Mrs. Fritz admits that she and her husband have not talked with Mark about sex. "We don't know what to tell him because of his birth defect." His father has told him the changes "are part of growing up and becoming a man." Mrs. Fritz is concerned because Mark "hasn't asked any questions like the other boys." (Mark is Tanner Stage 3.) "I think his brothers have talked with him because they joke around about making out."

Environmental Assessment

Familial. *Structure:* Mark is the youngest of three boys. Mrs. Fritz works part-time as a secretary and is home in the afternoon when Mark returns from school. Mr. Fritz works as a manger of a large department store. The grandparents (mother's side of the family) live nearby. The grandmother visits frequently. *Dynamics:* Mark is included in all family activities, and Mark and his brothers are involved in home activities and chores. It appears that the parents do not fully discuss all aspects of Mark's illness (sexuality issues, compliance, approaching adolescence) nor do they discuss all issues with Mark. The mother is overresponsible for Mark's treatments; she encourages Mark's overdependency. In turn, the mother assumes more responsibility for care.

Social/cultural. Mark is part of a Protestant, middle-class family who does not attend church regularly. Both parents place a high value on home and family. The father has assumed the patriarchal provider role in the family. The family has lived in the same house for 17 years and has several close friends in the neighborhood who will help whenever needed.

The parents have also maintained social relationships with several of Mr. Fritz's business associates. They belong to no outside social clubs or groups. Insurance covers 90% of Mark's expenses and financially "things are troublesome at times." Currently, there are no major financial problems.

Developmental. Mark laughed when I said he was about to become a "terrible teen." He said he has heard adults talk about it but he would not elaborate. Mark enjoys heavy metal rock, computer games, and watching television. When asked about girls, he shrugged and looked away. Mark attends a special education school and is behind grade level. His social skills are not age appropriate. Medical treatments, parental overprotectiveness, and physical disability all seem to be reinforcing dependence while diminishing any sense of self-control over health. Self-care responsibility is less than we would expect of a 12 year old.

Pathological and biological. Mark stated that he "hates everything about hospitals." He acknowledged that the increase in restrictions of activity bothered him. The "tests" and "surgery" worry him. He knows the surgery is to try to stop the "leaking" of urine, but Mark is unclear about where they will operate and exactly what will be done. Mark "doesn't like" diabetes because he can no longer "eat whatever I want." Mark has a poor understanding of diabetes. He could not explain the role of insulin and diet in the management of the illness. Mark has a better understanding of myelomeningocele and how that affects his walking and bowel and bladder control. On admission Mark's vital signs are normal. He is in the 25th percentile for height for his age and 90th percentile for weight. His BUN, creatinine, and blood sugar levels are slightly elevated. His glyohemoglobin level is elevated and indicates poor long-term control.

Ecological. The family owns a home in the suburbs. There is a park about a mile from home. There is a school and playground about one-half mile from home. The parents describe the neighborhood as safe. There is no public transportation available in the area.

Psychological. As a preadolescent, Mark is concerned about body image and anxious about any bodily disruption or change. He seems self-conscious about his early sexual maturation. His mother has noted Mark's childlike behaviors and increasing dependency during the past year (wants help dressing). He is socially isolated from peers, and interaction with his brothers has decreased during the past 2 years. There is also an increased need for more emotional support from his mother. Mark is described as shy by his mother and the nursing staff and my observations support this assessment. His scores on the self-esteem interview were low. He copes by withdrawing from situations that make him uncomfortable. He does not like to discuss his feelings about sensitive issues (parents, sexuality, illness). However, he wants information about specific events that are stressful for him (surgery).

• • •

This case study is presented because it reflects both acute and long-term problems associated with managing a chronic illness. It also demonstrates that children's developmental domains (behavioral subsystems) are often significantly influenced by their illness. One of the strengths of JBSM is that it not only identifies current acute problems but also identifies chronic subsystem alterations that are leading to behavioral system disturbances. These alterations involve a disturbance in normal developmental sequences. If there is no intervention, these alterations may lead to more serious problems as the child matures. This analysis will apply the nursing process to an acute problem related to this admission and to a long-term problem.

Diagnostic Analysis

The essential characteristic of human beings is their purposefulness. This purposefulness is based on their ability to select their goals and make choices for achieving them. To successfully intervene in a clinical situation, it is necessary to consider what people do and it is also necessary to understand why people make the choices they do. The JBSM directs the nurse's attention to human choice phenomena. The degree to which the nurse can help the person/client restore behavioral system balance depends on the extent to which behavioral actions are understood and can be explained. Once such an explanation has been found, behavioral system balance can be obtained by changing the goals that a person has or by changing the environmental conditions in such a way that previously established goals can be obtained through changes in behavior. To accomplish this, nurses need to adopt an input-oriented approach to their case-model building. To focus on the proper inputs, nurses need to develop an assessment strategy that allows them to understand small segments of behavior at the subsystem level thoroughly and then integrate that understanding for the entire system.

An output-oriented approach describes only the choices the person makes, and the description provides only knowledge of the behavior. This information is of some use. However, to understand the behavioral elements in the system, nurses must seek an explanation for a person's action, and this comes only from an input focus. The JBSM's focus on environmental assessment as well as behavioral assessment provides input-focused data as well as output-focused data. The two diagnoses addressed in this section provide insight about the process.

Acute problem. Mark has been admitted to the hospital for a bladder augmentation and placement of an artificial sphincter. He is behind in grade level at school. Piagetian testing places him at the concrete operations level of cognitive development. The subjective data inform the nurse that Mark is worried about "tests" and "surgery" and is unclear about specific aspects of the surgery. He has some understanding of myelomeningocele and little understanding about diabetes. However, he does like to have "tests and things" explained to him. Also contributing to this problem is the mother's overprotection of Mark and the apparent failure of the family to openly discuss aspects of the illness.

The goal of the ingestive subsystem is to internalize the external environment, and one of the functions is to obtain knowledge or information useful to the self (Grubbs, 1974). The perseveratory set refers to usual status or habits. All of Mark's sensory modalities—speech, sight, hearing and touch—are intact, and he values being informed about tests. In terms of the preparatory set, Mark is in the period of concrete operations. He can assimilate new experiences, has developed an awareness of conservation, is capable of seeing relationships of the part to the whole, and has also developed a concept of causality. Choice refers to the alternate behaviors Mark sees himself as being able to use in this situation. Since little preoperative teaching has been done, Mark's choice is limited as would be his actions. The diagnosis is insufficiency of the ingestive subsystem. The major stressor is functional—a lack of information. The nurse's goal is to protect the basic goal of the subsystem by providing information. A successful intervention will inform Mark about the surgery and the range of choices and actions will be clear.

Planning and Intervention

Given the complexity of this case, the intervention needs to be carefully planned. The intervention could also have an impact on the dependency subsystem (self-care), achievement subsystem (sense of mastery), affiliative subsystem (socialization), and eliminative subsystem (expression of feelings). It was mutually agreed that the preoperative teaching would be done with both Mark and his parents and alone with Mark. Diagrams and pictures would be used to explain the surgery, and postoperative treatments and procedures would also be explained and demonstrated. Thus the nurse will provide the functional requirements of protection and nurturance.

The immediate goal of the intervention is to inform Mark about the surgery and the postoperative care he will experience. The intermediate goal is that in the postoperative period Mark will maintain his health physiological system through the intake of food, fluids, and medicine. This will occur as a result of his understanding of the surgical procedure and the postoperative care needed for recovery (e.g., Mark is able to internalize the external environment). The long-term objective is that the intervention will begin to restore Mark's sense of mastery and his sense of autonomy.

Nursing interventions need to be theory based. These theories need to be compatible with systems theory and the assumptions of the JBSM. For example, the technique selected for this intervention is based on Vygotsky's zone of proximal development (ZPD) (Vygotsky, 1962). One of the strengths of the JBSM is the ease with which theories can be incorporated into all phases of the plan of care.

Wertsch and Rogoff (1984) have defined the ZPD as "the phase in development in which the child has only partially mastered a task but can participate in its execution with assistance and supervision of an adult or more capable peer" (p. 1). There are two important dimensions of the ZPD—joint collaboration and transfer of responsibility—in which both child and the adult actively participate and contribute to some aspect of task performance or problem solution. Joint collaboration is based on the child being guided to actively define and redefine the task situation in terms of the adult's definition (Holaday, LaMontagne, & Marciel, 1994).

The second dimension is the transfer of responsibility, which refers to the adult's decreasing role in regulating and managing behavior task performance. This gradual relinquishment and transfer of adult responsibility is described as "guided participation" (Wertsch & Rogoff, 1984). Thus, as a child's competence increases, effective scaffolders gradually withdraw their support in accord with the child's efforts. Scaffolding refers to the gradual decrease and eventual withdrawal of adult control and support as a function of the child's increasing mastery of a given task or problem.

Thus the preoperative teaching plan developed by the nurse, as an external regulator, for Mark is a scaffold. The nurse structures the situation but Mark makes decisions about his degree of involvement in the program and later about his role in postoperative care. Mark is supported and rewarded for his independent actions and efforts to regulate his care. This intervention also permits the nurse to role-model new behaviors for the parents.

Chronic problem. When the JBSM is used, it is helpful to think of parenting as a set of environmental actions performed by the parents or a set of environmental conditions arranged by parents that assists or impedes the child in carrying out his/her functions. It is important to make clear that in this examination of parenting actions and conditions as elements external to the child, the independence of the child and environment are not implied. Rather the examination is done only for the purposes of assessment and the convenience of organization.

From a JBSM perspective, the idea of an external regulator of growth and development is also useful. The idea of nursing care as a set of regulatory acts aimed at successful adaptation and goal attainment for the child (behavioral system) is consistent with most ecological developmental models and with the general precepts of control systems theory. However, as potentially useful as the concept of an external regulator might be as an organizing principle for classifying the actions and conditions of nursing care (i.e., in terms of adjusting parenting actions or environmental conditions arranged by the parent), it carries with it a practical paradox: external regulation is unlikely to be a simple matter for a complex organism. The JBSM provides a means to approach this issue, but we have a long way to go in building theory in this area. The next care problem clearly addresses the complexity involved.

The data from the environmental assessment identify Mark's mother as being overprotective and as assuming a high degree of responsibility for Mark's care. Mark spends a good deal of time with his mother and seems to be emotionally more attached to her than to his father. Mark is taking little responsibility for self-care activities. He is described as shy and cannot name a friend. The goal of the dependency subsystem is to maintain environmental resources needed for obtaining help, assistance, attention, reassurance, and security; in other words, to gain trust and reliance. The primary diagnosis is dominance of the dependency subsystem. The behaviors in the dependency subsystem are being used more than any other subsystem regardless of the situation and to the detriment of other subsystems (Grubbs, 1974). A number of secondary diagnoses could also be made in terms of incompatibility between the dependency subsystem (set, choice, action, and goal) and other subsystems (most notably achievement and affiliative). Problems for both child and parent are evident in terms of set, choice, and action. In terms of the perseveratory set, both parents and child are unclear about the appropriate age at which a child with a chronic health problem should be expected to meet their own needs and at which times and places should assistance with tasks be sought. Mark lacks a perception of himself as a self-sufficient and independent person. When the preparatory set is examined, it is clear that Mark and his parents have difficulty perceiving which situation is one in which task-oriented assistance is required and which is not. Given the problems with set, it is not surprising that the range of choice is narrow and actions are not always appropriate.

The major stressors are both functional and structural. The functional stressors arise from the environment and are related to parenting style. The structural stressors involve internal control mechanisms and reflect inconsistencies between the subsystem goal and set, choice, and action.

The short-term goals in this case are to help the parents gain some insight into their behavior and its impact on Mark's behavior and to facilitate a change in Mark's behavior (an increase in independent behaviors while hospitalized). The long-term goal is to promote Mark's optimal development by designing an external regulatory system to (1) sustain Mark's current level of independence, (2) stimulate activity directed at more independent behaviors, and (3) control the amount and pattern of experience (inputs) that reach Mark so there is an optimal fit between Mark's current abilities and his projected goals. This intervention would be best carried out by a nurse with sustained contact with Mark and his parents. This would be a family-centered intervention.

The central goal for the nurse, as an external regulatory force, is to construct a system of caregiving episodes for the parents that will be useful in integrating the functional requirements for the environmental/developmental relationship. The nurse would help the parents provide protection and nurturance to maintain Mark's current level of behavior (his internal organizational coherence and environmental relationships) so that Mark can continue to function. The nurse maintains whatever stability is present to avoid encouraging more dependent behaviors. The nurse stimulates incremental change (alter set, choice, and action) for both the parents and Mark through a process of self-construction. New information and new experiences will be introduced in a controlled fashion, which will lead to successive changes in existing structures. Goal setting is one technique that can be used to accomplish this. People have the ability to cognitively construct representations of potential future states. By personal goal setting, individuals disrupt their status quo or disorganize themselves and then organize their behavior to try to resolve the disruption or create a new coherent organization. They become "producers of their own development" (Lerner, 1982, p. 342). Thus in goal setting, negative feedback operates to reduce a discrepancy, but it does so by altering the system through incremental change.

Evaluation

The JBSM directs the nurse's attention toward areas that need to be addressed in practice. At present there is no specific intervention delineating this system of caregiving episodes for parents of chronically ill children. What broad, basic regulatory functions of the nurse need to be included in this system of caregiving episodes? The actual episodes and conditions of parenting entail numerous physical/structural properties, not just broad abstractions. The question is, from the standpoint of understanding the development of a chronically ill child, what are the most salient dimensions of these real acts and conditions for each of the subsystems? How does the nurse function as an external regulator of chronically ill children's health and development with the goal of "goodness of fit" between the child's characteristics, environmental opportunities, and constraints? In using the JBSM, the nurse learns that a chronically ill child's developmental pathways do not unfold along a predetermined course; they are constructed through processes of living that involve continuities, discontinuities, and uncertainties. The nurse as an external regulator and source of functional requirements plays a critical role in helping a family achieve optimal development outcomes for a special-needs child.

CRITICAL THINKING EXERCISES

1. Considering the assessment of Debbie according to the achievement subsystem, how might different goals (drive) or set have altered her choices or action? How would this difference have altered the structure of Debbie as a behavioral system?
2. What other two subsystems would have been altered by different goals or set? How might these different goals alter the structure of Debbie's behavioral system?
3. Think back to the last health problem you experienced. Recall your behaviors and assess their structure (drive, set, choice, and action) according to the behavioral assessment of the subsystems as outlined in Table 4-1.
4. Recall your environment at the time of your illness and assess your sustenal imperatives using the guide in Table 4-1.
5. Based on the assessments carried out in critical thinking exercises 3 and 4 above, conduct a diagnostic analysis on the data and determine what nursing diagnosis might have been used to guide the planning of nursing interventions for you according to Johnson's behavioral systems model.

References

Auger, J. (1976). *Behavioral systems and nursing.* Englewood Cliffs, NJ: Prentice-Hall.

Auger, J., & Dee, V. (1983). A patient classification system based on the Behavioral System Model of Nursing: Part 1. *Journal of Nursing Administration, 13*(4), 38-43.

Dee, V. (1990). Implementation of the Johnson model: One hospital's experience. In M. E. Parker (Ed.), *Nursing theories in practice* (pp. 33-44). New York: National League for Nursing.

Dee, V., & Randell, B. (1989). *NPH patient classification system: A theory-based nursing practice model for staffing.* Los Angeles: Nursing Department, UCLA Neuropsychiatric Institute and Hospital.

Derdiarian, A. K. (1983). An instrument for theory and research development using the behavioral system model for nursing: The cancer patient. Part I. *Nursing Research, 32,* 196-201.

Derdiarian, A. K. (1988). The sensitivity of the DBSM instrument to age, site and stage of cancer: A preliminary validation study. *Scholarly Inquiry for Nursing Practice, 2,* 103-120.

Derdiarian, A. K. (1990). The relationships among the subsystems of Johnson's behavioral system model. *Image: Journal of Nursing Scholarship, 22,* 219-225.

Derdiarian, A. K. (1993). The Johnson behavioral system model: Perspectives for nursing practice. In M. E. Parker (Ed.), *Patterns of Nursing Theories in Practice* (pp. 267-284). New York: National League for Nursing.

Derdiarian, A. K., & Forsythe, A. W. (1983). An instrument for theory and research development using the behavioral system model for nursing: The cancer patient. Part II. *Nursing Research, 32,* 260-266.

Glennin, C. G. (1980). Formulation of standards for nursing practice using a nursing model. In J. P. Riehl & C. Roy (Eds.), *Conceptual models for nursing practice,* (2nd ed., pp. 290-301). New York: Appleton-Century-Crofts.

Grubbs, J. (1974). The Johnson's behavioral system model. In J. Riehl & C. Roy (Eds.), *Conceptual Models for Nursing Practice* (pp. 217-249). New York: Appleton-Century-Croft.

Holaday, B. (1974). Achievement behavior in chronically ill children. *Nursing Research, 23,* 25-30.

Holaday, B. (1980). Implementing the Johnson model for nursing practice. In J. P. Riehl & C. Roy (Eds.), *Conceptual Models for Nursing Practice* (2nd ed., pp. 255-263). New York: Appleton-Century-Crofts.

Holaday, B. (1981). Maternal response to their chronically ill infants' attachment behavior of crying. *Nursing Research, 30,* 343-348.

Holaday, B. (1982). Maternal conceptual set development: Identifying patterns of maternal response to chronically ill infant crying. *Maternal Child Nursing Journal, 11*(1): 47-59.

Holaday, B. (1987). Patterns of interaction between mothers and their chronically ill infants. *Maternal Child Nursing Journal, 16,* 29-36.

Holaday, B., LaMontague, L., & Marciel, J. (1994). Vygotsky's zone of proximal development: Implications for nurse assistance of children's learning. *Issues in Comprehensive Pediatric Nursing, 17,* 15-27.

Holaday, B., Turner-Hensen, A., & Swan, J. (in press). *Explaining activities of chronically ill children: An analysis using the Johnson behavioral system model.* New York: National League for Nursing.

Johnson, D. (1968). *One conceptual model for nursing.* Paper presented at Vanderbilt University, Nashville, TN.

Johnson, D. (1980). The behavioral systems model for nursing. In J. Riehl & C. Roy (Eds.), *Conceptual Models for Nursing Practice,* (2nd ed., pp. 207-216). New York: Appleton-Century-Croft.

Johnson, D. (1990). The behavioral system model for nursing. In M. E. Parker (Ed.), *Nursing theories in practice,* (pp. 23-32). New York: National League for Nursing.

Lerner, R. M. (1982). Children and adolescents as producers of their own development. *Developmental Review, 2,* 342-370.

Majeslty, S. J., Brester, M. H., & Nishio, K. T. (1978). Development of a research tool: Patient indicators of nursing care. *Nursing Research, 27,* 365-371.

Meleis, A. I. (1991). *Theoretical nursing: Development and progress.* Philadelphia: J. B. Lippincott.

Pressley, M. (1992). Encouraging mindful use of prior knowledge: Attempting to construct explanatory answers facilitates learning. *Educational Psychologist, 27,* 91-109.

Rawls, A. G. (1980). Evaluation of the Johnson behavioral model in clinical practice. *Image, 12,* 13-16.

Riegel, B. (1989). Social support and psychological adjustment to chronic coronary heart disease: Operationalization of Johnson's behavioral system model. *Advances in Nursing Science, 11*(2): 74-84.

Vygotsky, L. S. (1962). *Thought and language.* Cambridge, MA: MCT Press.

Weisman, A. D. (1979). *Coping with cancer.* New York: McGraw-Hill.

Wertsch, J. V., & Rogoff, B. (1984). Editor's notes. *New Directions for Child Development, 23,* 1-6.

Wittrock, M. C. (1990). Generative processes of comprehension. *Educational Psychologist, 24,* 345-376.

King's Systems Framework and Theory in Nursing Practice

Maureen A. Frey and Diane Norris

"Knowledge used by nurses has been derived from natural and behavioral sciences. More recently, nurses have been discussing nursing science and studying ways in which an organized body of knowledge essential to nursing practice can be identified." (King, 1968)

HISTORY AND BACKGROUND

In the mid-1960s, Imogene King wrote of the need for focus, organization, and use of nursing's knowledge base (King, 1968). Knowledge for nursing results from the systematic use and validation of knowledge about concepts relevant to nursing situations. In discussing the role of concepts in knowledge development, King stated, "Concepts offer a way of thinking about nursing: a way of observing behavior and a way of collecting specific information essential for decision making based on knowledge available to meet some of the needs of individuals at a particular point in time" (p. 30). Use of knowledge in practice leads to the generating and testing of hypotheses.

In 1971, King proposed a conceptual frame of reference for nursing around four concepts she believed to be universal to the discipline of nursing: social systems, health, perception, and interpersonal relationships. These areas were identified from synthesis and reformulation using inductive and deductive reasoning, critical thinking, and extensive review of nursing and other literature. The concepts were organized around individuals as personal systems, small groups as interpersonal systems, and larger social systems such as community and school (King, 1971). Role, status, social organization, communication, information, and energy were identified as basic concepts of functions of systems. King proposed that the concepts were interrelated and could be used across systems with a goal of identifying the essence of nursing.

King expanded the conceptual framework during the 1970s by further explicating the nature of persons and environment, strengthening the general systems orientation, and expanding the concepts. A more formalized conceptual framework of personal, interpersonal, and social systems was presented by King in 1981. Concepts in the personal system were perception, self, growth and development, body image, time, and space. Concepts in the interpersonal system were human interaction, communication, transactions, role, and stress. Concepts in the social system were organization, authority, power, status, and decision making.

Also presented in the 1981 text was the theory of goal attainment. This theory specifically addressed how nurses interact with patients to achieve health goals. Initially, the concepts of the theory, derived from the personal and interpersonal systems, were perception, communication, interaction, transaction, stress, growth and development, self, role, time, and space (King, 1981). Since 1981, King has provided clarification, explanation, and some additional expansion of concepts. The concepts of learning and coping were added, the concept of space was redefined as personal space, and the concept of stress was expanded to include stressors (Frey, in press; King, 1990, 1991). In addition, King has addressed issues raised by others who analyzed her framework (e.g., Gonot 1989; Fawcett, 1989; Magan, 1987; Meleis, 1991) as have Carter and Dufour (1994). There has also been a dramatic increase in the number of publications based on King's framework and theory as well as other theories derived from the systems framework. In 1995, the first text devoted solely to the advancement and application of King's framework and theory was published (Frey & Sieloff, 1995).

OVERVIEW OF KING'S SYSTEMS FRAMEWORK AND THEORY

King's systems framework for nursing consists of concepts organized around personal, interpersonal, and social systems. According to King (1981, 1988, 1991), concepts are critical because it is knowledge about concepts that is applied in practice. Concepts are defined as follows.

Personal Systems

Perception: "Process of organizing, interpreting, and transforming information from sense data and memory" (King, 1981, p. 24).

Self: "The self is a composite of thoughts and feelings which constitute a person's awareness of his/her individual existence, his/her conception of who and what he/she is. A person's self is the sum total of all he/she can call his/hers. The self includes among other things, a system of ideas, attitudes, values and commitments. The self is a person's total subjective environment. It is a distinctive center of experience and significance. The self constitutes a person's inner world as distinguished from the outer world consisting of all other people and things. The self is the individual as known to the individual. It is that to which we refer when we say 'I'" (Jersild, 1952, pp. 9-10, cited in King, 1981, p. 28).

Growth and development: "The processes that take place in an individual's life that help the individual move from potential capacity for achievement to self-actualization" (King, 1981, p. 31).

Body image: "An individual's perceptions of his/her own body, others' reactions to his/her appearance which results from others' reactions to self" (King, 1981, p. 33).

Learning: "A process of sensory perception, conceptualization, and critical thinking involving multiple experiences in which changes in concepts, skills, symbols, habits, and values can be evaluated in observable behaviors and inferred from behavioral manifestation" (King, 1986, p. 24).

Time: "Duration between the occurrence of one event and occurrence of another event" (King, 1981, p. 24).

Personal space: "Existing in all directions and is the same everywhere" (King, 1981, p. 37).

Coping: "The constantly changing cognitive and behavioral efforts to manage specific external and internal demands that are appraised as taxing or exceeding the resources" (Lazarus & Folkman, 1984, p. 141). Note: King did not define the concept of coping. The use of Lazarus and Folkman's definition is suggested by Doornbos (1995).

Interpersonal Systems

Communication: "Information processing, a change of information from one state to another" (King, 1981, p. 69).

Interaction: "Acts of two or more persons in mutual presence" (King, 1981, p. 85).

Role: "Set of behaviors expected when occupying a position in a social system" (King, 1981, p. 93).

Stress: "Dynamic state whereby a human being interacts with the environment to maintain balance for growth, development, and performance which involves an exchange of energy and information between the person and the environment for regulation and control of stressors" (King, 1981, p. 98).

Stressors: Events that produce stress (based on the definition of stress).

Transaction: "Observable behaviors of human beings interacting with their environment" (King, 1981, p. 147).

Social Systems

Organization: "A system whose continuous activities are conducted to achieve goals" (King, 1981, p. 119).

Authority: "Transactional process characterized by active, reciprocal relations in which members' values, backgrounds, and perceptions play a role in defining, validating, and accepting the [directions] of individuals within an organization" (King, 1981, p. 124).

Power: "Capacity to use resources in organizations to achieve goal . . . process whereby one or more persons influence other persons in a situation . . . capacity or ability of a group to achieve goals" (King, 1981, p. 124).

Status: "The position of an individual in a group or a group in relation to other groups in an organization" (King, 1981, p. 129).

Decision making: "Dynamic and systematic process by which a goal-directed choice of perceived alternatives is made, and acted upon, by individuals or groups to answer a question and attain a goal" (King, 1981, p. 132).

The framework provides both structure and function for nursing. Clearly stated assumptions about persons, environment, health, nursing, and systems provide a conceptual orientation of holism and dynamic interaction, identify health as the goal of nursing, and actively include the patient (individual, family, or community) in decisions about setting and working toward health goals.

The theory of goal attainment specifically addresses nursing as a process of human interaction. Concepts in the theory of goal attainment are perception, communication, interaction, transaction, self, role, growth and development, stress/stressors, coping, time, and personal space. King (1981, 1991) identified that perception, communication, and interaction are essential elements in transaction, but transactions cannot be directly observed; rather they are inferred based on the presence of the following elements of interaction: action, reaction, disturbance, mutual goal setting, exploring means to achieve goals, and agreeing on means to attain them. When transactions are made, goals are usually attained. The human interaction and conceptual focus dimensions of the theory guide the nursing process dimension as illustrated in Figure 5-1.

King has demonstrated the link between the theory of goal attainment and nursing process as shown in Table 5-1 (King, 1992). King (1993) views the nursing process as a system of interrelated actions. The nurse and client are an interpersonal system in which each affects the other and both are affected by situational factors. Nursing process is the vehicle through which nursing is practiced. The structure of the nursing process is assess, plan, implement, and evaluate. The content is informed by knowledge of the concepts in the systems framework.

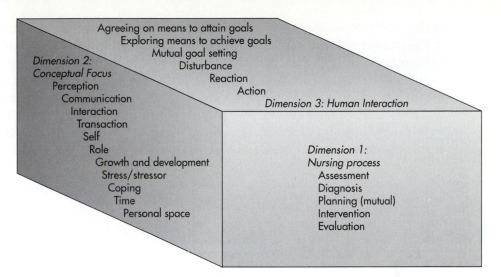

FIGURE 5-1

Three-dimensional nursing process based on King's theory. (Modified from Alligood, M. R. [1995]. Theory of goal attainment: Application to adult orthopedic nursing. In M. A. Frey & C. L. Sieloff [Eds.], *Advancing King's systems framework and theory for nursing* [p. 212]. Thousand Oaks, CA: Sage Publications.)

TABLE 5-1 Nursing Process: Theory and Method	
Nursing Process as Method*	**Nursing Process as Theory†**
A system of interrelated actions	A system of interrelated concepts
Assess	Perception of nurse and client
	Communication of nurse and client
	Interaction of nurse and client
Plan	Decision making about goals
	Agree to means to attain goals
Implement	Transactions made
Evaluate	Goal attained (if not, why not)

From King, I. M. (1992). King's theory of goal attainment. *Nursing Science Quarterly, 5*(1), 23.
*Yura, H., & Walsh, M. (1983). *The nursing process.* Norwalk, CT: Appleton-Century-Crofts.
†King, I. M. (1981). *A theory for nursing: Systems, concepts, process.* New York: John Wiley. (Now published by Delmar, Albany, NY).

CRITICAL THINKING IN NURSING PRACTICE WITH KING'S FRAMEWORK

It is generally agreed that critical thinking is knowing how: how to think, how to apply, how to analyze, how to synthesize, and how to evaluate. Whereas the nursing process of assess, plan, implement, and evaluate provides a method, the critical thinking process emphasizes intellectual skills of apprehension, judgment, and reasoning. According to Doona (1992), nursing has only recently begun to focus attention on critical thinking skills. However, the process of decision making in nursing situations requires critical thinking, which has always been an integral component in King's perspective of nursing. One of the strongest elements linking critical thinking to nursing practice is King's emphasis on the mental acts of judgment that are implicit in perception, communication, and interactions that lead to transaction (King, 1992). Actually, in her early writing, King (Daubenmire & King, 1973) presented a diagram (Figure 5-2) titled "methodology for the study of nursing process."

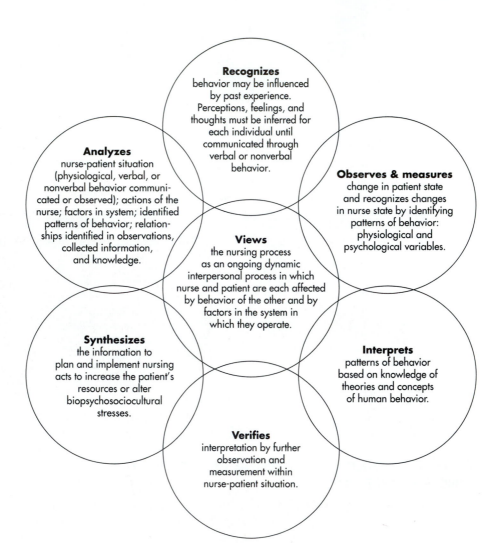

FIGURE 5-2

Methodology for the study of the nursing process. (From Daubenmire, M. J., & King, I. M. [1973]. Nursing process: A system approach. *Nursing Outlook, 21*[8], 515.)

Critical thinking is evident in this early work by the use of terms such as *analyze, synthesize, verify,* and *interpret.*

The interface of the nursing process as interrelated actions, the critical-thinking process as highly developed thinking skills, and the transaction process, which includes knowledge of the concepts contained in the general systems framework and knowledge of professional interactions as identified in the theory of goal attainment, is shown in Table 5-2.

• • •

Use of critical thinking and nursing process as a method related to transactions is demonstrated in the following case of Debbie.

TABLE 5-2	Relationship Among the Three Processes	
Nursing Process	**Critical Thinking Process**	**Transaction Process**
Assess and apply knowledge of relevant concepts	Conceptualize	Client and nurse perceive each other and situation, make judgments, mental actions, and reactions
		Interaction is an ongoing process characterized by communication
		The nurse:
		Gathers additional information
		Validates perceptions
		Delineates and validates patient concerns
		Establishes mutuality and trust
Identify goals and plans to achieve	Analyze/ synthesize	Make decisions about goals
		Goal must be considered in light of capabilities and limitations of patient
		Goals must be mutually set
		Decisions for actions to meet goals
Implement actions to meet goals		Transactions made
		Not directly observed
		Inferred from interactions
Evaluate goal attainment	Evaluate	Goals attained; if not, why not?
		Unmet goals can result from:
		Identification of incorrect or incomplete data
		Incorrect interpretation as the result of perceptual error, lack of knowledge, or goal conflict
		Contributing nurse, patient, system barriers

ASE HISTORY OF DEBBIE

Debbie is a 29-year-old woman who was recently admitted to the oncology nursing unit for evaluation after sensing pelvic "fullness" and noticing a watery, foul-smelling vaginal discharge. A Papanicolaou smear revealed a class V cervical cancer. She was found to have a stage II squamous cell carcinoma of the cervix and underwent a radical hysterectomy with bilateral salpingooophorectomy.

Her past health history revealed that physical examinations had been infrequent. She also reported that she had not performed breast self-examination. She is 5 feet 4 inches tall and weighs 89 pounds. Her usual weight is about 110 pounds. She has smoked approximately two packs of cigarettes a day for the past 16 years. She is gravida 2, para 2. Her first pregnancy was at age 16, and her second was at age 18. Since that time she has taken oral contraceptives on a regular basis.

Debbie completed the eighth grade. She is married and lives with her husband and two children in her mother's home, which she describes as less than sanitary. Her husband is unemployed. She describes him as emotionally distant and abusive at times.

She has done well following surgery except for being unable to completely empty her urinary bladder. She is having continued postoperative pain and nausea. It will be necessary for her to perform intermittent self-catheterization at home. Her medications are (1) an antibiotic, (2) an analgesic as needed for pain, and (3) an antiemetic as needed for nausea. In addition, she will be receiving radiation therapy on an outpatient basis.

Debbie is extremely tearful. She expresses great concern over her future and the future of her two children. She believes that this illness is a punishment for her past life.

NURSING CARE OF DEBBIE WITH KING'S FRAMEWORK

From King's framework, Debbie is conceptualized as a personal system in interaction with other systems. Many of these interactions influence her health. In addition, her recent diagnosis of class V cervical cancer influences her health. Together Debbie and the nurse communicate, engage in mutual goal setting, and make decisions about the means to achieve goals.

Nursing care for Debbie begins with assessment, which includes collection, interpretation, and verification of data. Sources of data are Debbie herself, primarily perception, behavior, and past experiences; knowledge of concepts in the systems framework; critical thinking skills; ability to use nursing process; and medical knowledge about the treatment and prognosis of class V cervical cancer. Care for Debbie may well cover the full range of nursing practice: promotion of health, maintenance and restoration of health, care of the sick, and care of the dying (King, 1981).

In nursing situations, the nurse forms an interpersonal system with Debbie. The transaction process begins with perception, judgments, mental actions, and reactions of both individuals. The nurse assesses and applies knowledge of concepts and processes. Although all of the concepts in King's framework will likely contribute to the nursing care of Debbie, critical concepts are perception, self, coping, interaction, role, stress, power, and decision making.

The nurse's perception serves as a basis for gathering and interpreting information. Debbie's perceptions influence her thoughts and actions and are assessed through verbal and nonverbal behaviors. Because perceptual accuracy is important to the interaction process, the nurse validates her own perceptions and her interpretation of Debbie's perceptions with Debbie. Debbie's perceptions might be influenced by her emotional state, stress, or pain. The nurse's perceptions are influenced by culture, socioeconomic status, age, and diagnosis of the patient (King, 1981). Perceptions form the basis for development of the self.

According to King (1981), self is the conception of who and what one is and includes one's subjective totality of attitudes, values, experiences, commitments, and awareness of individual existence. Debbie reveals important information about self. She is tearful and expresses fear, concern, uncertainty, and blame. Her past behavior provides some basis for her present feeling in that Debbie has not taken actions to promote and maintain her own health.

Clearly, feelings about self and situation are psychological stressors. Debbie has physical and interpersonal stressors as well. Physical stressors are a result of the illness and surgery. Bladder function, pain, and nausea are identified as immediate problems, and radiation treatment may result in other changes in physical status. In the interpersonal system, Debbie identifies a distant and often abusive relationship with her husband, which is a major lack of emotional support during this very difficult time. Since he is unemployed and she is unable to work, lack of money and other basic resources are likely to be stressors as well. Her husband's inability to provide basic emotional and material support most likely contributes to Debbie's concern for her children, especially with changes that are likely to occur in her own role with them. An additional stressor is the living situation. In addition to being unsanitary, it seems quite crowded. Debbie's perception of the situation needs additional assessment as it might only be the nurse's perception that her home situation will interfere with necessary postoperative care. It is also possible that the lack of personal, and perhaps family, space contributes to stress. Coping with personal and interpersonal stressors is likely to influence both health and illness outcomes. Debbie may need additional resources to help her cope with the immediate situation and the future.

Communication is the key to establishing mutuality and trust between Debbie and the nurse and the means to validating perceptions, establishing patient priorities, and moving the interaction process toward goal setting. Debbie is expected to participate in identifying goals. However, direction from the nurse will likely be necessary because of the overwhelming needs and lack of resources. Nurses can find direction for assisting patients to identify goals based on the assumptions that underlie King's systems framework. For example, the overall goal of nursing is to assist persons to function in their roles (King, 1981). Debbie has expressed major concerns about her children, which may involve the maternal role. However, Debbie is also in the patient role, one that may change based on the recovery process and/or progression or remission of cancer. Another basic assumption is that nurses assist patients to adjust to changes in their health status. Decisions about goals must be based on the capabilities, limitations, priorities of the patient, and situation. In this situation, the immediate goals seem to be control of postoperative pain and nausea, although this needs validation with Debbie. Debbie will also need to be able to perform self-catheterization when necessary at home.

It is not clear from the data available about Debbie to know if her fears, worries, and anxieties are interfering with her ability to participate in prioritizing goals or to identify or participate in actions to meet goals. But if they were, the first nursing action would be to obtain psychological assessment and crisis intervention as necessary. Other important goals and actions might be directed toward mobilizing resources, especially family support. Although Debbie's mother may not be a very good housekeeper, she may be a good source of emotional support and direct aid and service such as transportation for outpatient treatments. It is possible that professional goals and patient goals may be incongruent. Continuous analysis, synthesis, and validation are critical to keep on track.

In addition to decisions about goals, Debbie is expected to be involved in decisions about actions to meet goals. Involving Debbie in decision making may be a challenge because of her sense of powerlessness over the illness, treatment, and ability to contribute to family functioning. Yet empowering Debbie is likely to increase her sense of self, which in turn can reduce stress, improve coping, change perceptions, and lead to changes in her physical state.

Goal attainment needs ongoing evaluation. For Debbie, follow-up on pain, nausea, and bladder function soon after discharge will be necessary. One way to do this might be to arrange for in-home nursing services (a nursing action meeting a goal). Having a professional in the home would also contribute to further assessment of the family, validation of progress toward goals, and modifications in plans to achieve goals.

According to King, if transactions are made, goals will be attained. Goal attainment can improve or maintain health, control illness, or lead to a peaceful death. If goals are not attained, the nurse needs to reexamine the nursing process, critical-thinking process, and transaction process. Unmet goals can result from an incorrect or incomplete data base, perceptual errors, lack of knowledge, lack of mutuality in the relationship, goal conflict as well as any number of other nurse, patient, or system barriers (Kameoka, 1995).

• • •

A second example of the use of the theory of goal attainment is shown in the case of Clare, an infant in the neonatal intensive care unit (NICU) experiencing a complicated medical course and uncertain future. King's theory of goal attainment facilitates interactions that lead to transactions and progress toward goals for Clare and her family.

ASE HISTORY OF CLARE

Clare was born on March 31, 1995, by an elective cesarean section to a 33-year-old mother and 35-year-old father at 37 weeks' gestation. This was the mother's second pregnancy. She received prenatal care and both pregnancies were uneventful. The first child is a 6-year-old son who was hospitalized at birth and now has severe developmental delays. He requires constant care but is in a special program during the daytime hours.

At birth Clare weighed 3665 g (about 8 pounds) and had Apgar scores of 8 and 9, which indicated that she was in good condition at birth. However, respiratory distress developed several hours after birth. Clare was intubated and placed on a ventilator but required increasing amounts of oxygen and pressure with no improvement in blood gases. At 36 hours of age, she was transferred to a tertiary level NICU and within 2 hours of admission was placed on extracorporeal membrane oxygenation (ECMO). During the next few days, complications including sepsis, seizures, and renal failure arose. One or both of Clare's parents visited daily.

After 8 days Clare was doing well enough to be taken off ECMO but remained intubated on ventilator support. She was stable for the next 3 days but then began to require increased ventilator support to the point that survival was questionable. It was decided to place her on experimental nitrous oxide treatment for "compassionate" support since there were no other options to offer the family. Over the next few days, Clare's condition was very unstable with multiple episodes of "ups and downs."

The family, including the paternal grandparents, talked to the neonatologist about Clare's survival, the quality of her life if she survived, and any pain or discomfort she might be experiencing at present. They also discussed the possibility of organ donation. On the sixth day of nitrous oxide treatment her condition deteriorated even further and she was not expected to survive more than a few hours. The family asked for the hospital chaplain to perform an emergency baptism.

Amazingly Clare began to improve over the next few days although she remained on a ventilator. Then another setback occurred. It was necessary to insert chest tubes to drain fluid accumulation in her chest. However, a week later she was tolerating gavage feedings well although the chest tube remained in place. Blood gas levels continued to improve and Clare was eventually extubated. Her condition stabilized and she began to make steady progress. It was anticipated that Clare would be discharged to her family at some point in the future when her physiological problems were resolved and growth was adequate.

NURSING CARE OF CLARE WITH KING'S FRAMEWORK

On April 3, 1995, Anne Collins arrives for her day shift in the NICU and finds that she is assigned to Clare. Anne is asked to become Clare's primary nurse. Concepts that King (1981) articulates in her framework and theory of goal attainment provide a basis for critical thinking, which Anne uses during the process of caring for Clare and her family.

There are three time periods described in Clare's case study. The first phase covers the first 2 weeks when Clare was on ECMO and began to recover. The next period is a week's duration when it seemed likely that Clare would not survive. The last period describes a period of stabilization and progress toward eventual discharge. Only the first time period will be used to illustrate the use of King's work in nursing practice because of the complexity of the case.

The first step in the process is conceptualization and assessment using each of the concepts identified within each system. Anne begins to think about Clare and her family in terms of King's three interrelated systems: personal, interpersonal, and social. The personal system in King's framework refers to the individual. In Clare's case, Anne identifies four individuals, each comprising a personal system: Clare, her mother, her father, and Anne. Interpersonal systems are formed when two or more personal systems interact. Anne recognizes the presence of multiple interpersonal systems that may impact on Clare. Social systems are represented by larger groups, which influence the personal and interpersonal systems. Anne takes note of Clare's extended family, particularly her grandparents. She also thinks about religious systems that might play a role in Clare's case because Clare's survival is uncertain. Anne also recognizes that the NICU is a social system with its own inherent and often overwhelming power and authority, values, patterns of behavior, and role expectations.

One strongly held value in this NICU is the philosophy of family-centered care, which recognizes and respects the role of families in the care of their children. Anne is aware that some would challenge the usefulness of King's framework in caring for patients like Clare who are incapable of expressing themselves and participating in goal planning. However, Anne believes that King's framework is useful for nursing practice in a family-centered NICU because interactions, transactions, and mutual goal setting can be achieved in partnership with Clare's parents. These activities will promote the health of the family system, which is the goal of nursing in King's framework, by assisting Clare's parents to function in their roles as parents.

Now that Anne has conceptualized Clare and her family in terms of the three interacting systems, she gathers data and applies knowledge of the concepts identified within the personal system: perception, self, growth and development, body image, time, and personal space. Anne recognizes that most of these concepts do not apply to Clare as a newborn except that of growth and development. Anne knows that Clare's illness and its treatment will interfere with normal newborn behavior, which could impede parental interaction and possibly attachment to her. It is also possible that Clare will not meet developmental milestones, either on time or at all. It is likely that development will be less problematic for Clare at this point in her life than for her parents. The sense of chronic sorrow that accompanies the "loss" of a perfect, healthy infant for all parents may well be magnified for these parents because of their experiences with their son and his status.

Anne then turns her attention to concepts that are important in order to assess Clare's parents. Clare's father visited at least once a day and phoned often during the first four days of Clare's life, but Anne was not on duty when he visited. During that time he had to provide care for his son and support his wife who was recovering from a cesarean section.

Clare's parents visited together for the first time on the fourth day of her hospitalization. It was important to assess Clare's parents' perceptions of her health status and the situation. Clare's mother was very upset and sobbing; her father appeared overwhelmed. After providing them an opportunity to express their emotional tensions and grief, Anne engaged them in conversation about Clare. They expressed shock over the events following her birth. They had waited 6 years to have another child until their son was in school and they felt they could handle the demands of a newborn. Despite the health status of their son and the fact that no specific causes for his delays were ever identified, these parents had no reason to expect anything but a normal, healthy child this time. Both parents expressed concern for Clare's survival and also for any long-term health implications. Anne perceived that Clare's parents were exhibiting a normal, appropriate reaction to the present situation. Their perceptions of Clare's status were congruent with Anne's, were a fair estimation of the reality and uncertainty of the situation, and were clearly influenced by their past experience.

Another important concept is self. Clare's parents bring a unique "self" to this experience that defines them as individuals. Clare's parents already had established themselves as mother and father with their first-born. They also had 6 years of experience with their developmentally disabled son. Anne also considered the possibility that Clare's parents may be experiencing guilt and anger about having another child with major health problems because they repeatedly questioned what was the matter with them that they could not have a normal child.

The concept of personal space is pertinent in the care of Clare and her parents. There is no personal, private space in the NICU in which Clare's parents can express themselves, interact with Clare, or interact with others. There are four other infants in the same room with Clare. Furthermore, the space around Clare's warmer is congested because of the number of life support machines in use. The unit does have several screens that Anne uses to provide some small amount of privacy for short periods of time.

Time is another concept within the personal system that affects Clare's parents. Time represents a continuous flow of events, one after the other, which leads to the future. The uncertainty surrounding Clare's medical status requires continual adjustment in terms of time. Clare's parents kept asking when she would be able to be taken off ECMO. For her parents, that event represented movement toward the future, to survival. When she was finally taken off ECMO, her parents expected that in time she would be ready to go home. Unfortunately, this time sequence was disrupted by other life-threatening crises.

Growth and development is also a relevant concept for Clare's parents. The addition of another family member signals a development change: now the family unit is expanded to four. Clare's parents will continue to grow and develop as parents as they assimilate Clare into the family. This process might be challenged by the special needs of both children.

Pertinent concepts in the interpersonal system that Anne considers include interaction, communication, transaction, role, and stressors/stress. Throughout Clare's hospitalization, Anne communicates with Clare's parents and provides them with information that they need to function in their parental role. Open communication with Clare's parents enables Anne to validate their perceptions and judgments and understand their actions and reactions. Such communication establishes mutuality and trust between Anne and Clare's parents, which in turn leads to interactions and ultimately transactions. One characteristic of interactions is reciprocity, an interdependence in the relationship in which there is an exchange between the persons involved. Clare's mother regularly brought cookies or donuts for the nursing staff as her way of giving something back to the staff in exchange for their support and care of Clare and her family.

Anne recognizes that there are multiple psychological and social stressors inherent in the NICU experience that cause stress for Clare's parents. The uncertain outcome and prognosis of Clare's illness is a major one. Clare's parents verbalize that it is difficult to adjust to changes in Clare's condition. At one moment they feel hopeful; the next they feel despair. Other times they do not know what they hope the outcome will be.

The NICU itself is a noisy, bustling, tension-filled environment. All kinds of alarms and buzzers send out signals of potential disaster, which heighten concerns for Clare's parents. Clare's parents often comment on unexpected and unplanned stress in their day-to-day lives: they must continue to provide for their older son, they feel compelled to visit Clare daily, they must drive back and forth to the hospital, and must maintain the normal routines of washing, grocery shopping, and work.

Role is another important concept in the interpersonal system. Anne knows that parents often feel inadequate in their role as parents compared to the role of the nurse who cares for their infant. An alteration in parenting role may interfere with Clare's parents' ability to engage in mutual goal setting, which leads to transactions (Norris & Hoyer, 1993). Anne brings a strong commitment to family-centered care to her nursing practice. Initially she defines the goal of helping Clare's parents establish their role as Clare's parents and also plans to redefine that goal with Clare's parents when they are ready.

The concepts of authority, power, status, and decision making are characteristics of social systems that are relevant in Clare's case. Anne knows that the NICU represents a high-tech, threatening arena for most parents, unlike any other social situation they have experienced. As a social system, the NICU possesses authority and power that appears to exceed that of parents. Parents often perceive that they do not have much status. Physicians and nurses have expertise and skills with which parents cannot compete when it comes to caring for their child. Unless the NICU supports a philosophy of family-centered care, parents may not be actively involved in care or care decisions.

At one point Anne observed that Clare's mother had a tendency to focus on the details of the technological care being provided but Clare's father would tell her "not to sweat the small details." While Anne recognized that Clare's parents had different coping styles, she also perceived that Clare's mother may be feeling powerlessness in the present situation. In addition, Anne recognized that loss of control may threaten the self. Clare's mother may feel threatened and therefore make issues out of little things. Anne took an opportunity to discuss her perceptions with Clare's mother who validated that she did not feel like a mother. She said that there was nothing she could do for Clare as her mother because the nurses did everything.

Taken together, the concepts of interaction, perception, communication, transaction, self, role, stressors/stress, growth and development, time, and personal space constitute the theory of goal attainment. Through communication and interaction, Anne and Clare's parents clarified their perceptions of reality and mutually established the following goal: to identify aspects of care that they could provide within the constraints of Clare's physical condition and treatment. Anne's role was to teach and assist them to care for Clare safely. Within several days Anne observed that Clare's mother independently initiated aspects of care for Clare and was becoming adept at performing them even within the confined space. As Clare's mother's confidence in herself increased, she became less focused on minor changes in blood gas levels or ventilator settings and began to function in the role of parent of her infant in the NICU. Clare's mother demonstrated growth and development in behavioral activities related to parenting in the environment and social system of the NICU. Anne observed that verbal and nonverbal manifestations of stress decreased for both of Clare's parents.

The process of goal attainment occurs within the context of time, with one event leading to another. Discussion and clarification of perceptions leads to judgment, action, and reaction for both Anne and Clare's parents. These activities were followed by mutual establishment of goals during the process of interaction, which led to achievement of goals. Achievement of goals is transaction. Transactions lead to improved health—in this case, Clare's parents' ability to be parents to their infant.

Over time Clare's physical condition continued to improve to the point at which survival was likely but the need for special care when she goes home remained high. This represents a critical time for parental participation in goal setting and development of plans to meet those goals so that they would be prepared to assume full-time parenting roles and skills when they get home. For example, infants who have been on ECMO are often slow to establish bottle-feeding. Anne will communicate this information to Clare's parents to decrease potential stress caused by unrealistic expectations and coordinate a consultation with occupational therapy to teach Clare's parents feeding strategies that will promote adequate weight gain and growth.

The challenge to nurses working in the NICU is to look beyond the technological care they provide to the importance of interaction and transaction early in the hospitalization of a sick infant. Families expect that technological care will be appropriate and competent. In addition, they also need a caring relationship with nurses. As one mother put it when discussing her NICU experience with her son, "The facts of his history will remain the same. How we perceive the experience may be changed. The memories are tempered by the relationships we formed. In partnership, you will make a permanent, positive difference in the life in an NICU family" (Busch, 1992, p. 8).

King's theory of goal attainment (1981) provides direction for nursing practice in the NICU because it emphasizes the process of communication, interaction, and transactions, which is a foundation for promoting and maintaining health status of individuals and families (Norris & Hoyer, 1993). The relationships that nurses establish with parents based on mutual respect and trust also attain the goal of nursing, which is "to help individuals to maintain their health so that they can function in their roles" (King, 1981, pp. 4-5). Nurses who work with parents to mutually establish and attain goals will influence health outcomes of personal and interpersonal systems.

CRITICAL THINKING EXERCISES

1. Suggest two nursing diagnoses you would expect Anne to develop during this first phase of care. State two goals (assume they are mutually derived) and identify two specific nursing actions for each goal.
2. During the second and third phases of Clare's hospitalization, what additional information would Anne want to assess within each of King's systems?
3. Following discharge, Clare and her parents are seen in the developmental assessment clinic. Compare the concepts you would assess for Clare as a personal system when she is 2 years of age.
4. You are a senior in college and are sharing an apartment with two other students. Parents' weekend is 3 days away and all of your parents will be visiting the apartment for the first time. It has not been cleaned or straightened up since the beginning of the semester 8 weeks ago. Two weeks ago you all agreed that you wanted the apartment to look nice for your parents so they would be proud of you. Describe the personal, interpersonal, and social system factors that have contributed to your share of this mess! How will you achieve your goal over the next 3 days?

References

Busch, J. (1992). Partners in care: Parents and professionals in the NICU. *NANNews,5*(5), 1, 6-8.

Carter, K. F., & Dufour, L. T. (1994). King's theory: A critique of the critiques. *Nursing Science Quarterly,* 7(3), 128-133.

Daubenmire, M. J., & King, I. M. (1973). Nursing process: A system approach. *Nursing Outlook, 21*(8), 512-517.

Doona, M. E. (1992). Judgment: The nurse's key to knowledge. *Journal of Professional Nursing,* 8(4), 31-38.

Doornbos, M. M. (1995). Using King's systems framework to explore family health in the families of the young chronically mentally ill. In M. A. Frey & C. L. Sieloff (Eds.), *Advancing King's systems framework and theory of nursing* (pp. 192-205). Thousand Oaks, CA: Sage Publications.

Fawcett, J. (1989). *Analysis and evaluation of conceptual models.* Philadelphia: F. A. Davis.

Frey, M. A. (in press). King's systems framework for nursing. In J. Fitzpatrick & A. Whall (Eds.), *Conceptual models of nursing: Analysis and application* (3rd ed.). Norwalk, CT: Appleton & Lange.

Frey, M. A., & Sieloff, C. L. (1995). *Advancing King's systems framework and theory for nursing.* Thousand Oaks, CA: Sage Publications.

Gonot, P. W. (1989). Imogene King's conceptual framework of nursing. In J. Fitzpatrick & A. Whall (Eds.), *Conceptual models of nursing: Analysis and application* (2nd ed., pp. 271-283). Norwalk, CT: Appleton & Lange.

Kameoka, T. (1995). Analyzing nurse-patient interaction in Japan. In M. A. Frey & C. L. Sieloff (Eds.), *Advancing King's systems framework and theory for nursing.* Thousand Oaks, CA: Sage Publications.

King, I. M. (1968). A conceptual frame of reference. *Nursing Research, 17*(1), 27-31.

King, I. M. (1971). *Toward a theory for nursing.* New York: John Wiley.

King, I. M. (1981). *A theory for nursing: Systems, concepts, process.* New York: Delmar.

King, I. M. (1986). *Curriculum and instruction in nursing: Concepts and process.* Norwalk, CT: Appleton-Century-Crofts.

King, I. M. (1988). Concepts: Essential elements in theories. *Nursing Science Quarterly, 1*(1), 22-25.

King, I. M. (1990, July). *The theory of goal attainment: An update.* Paper presented at Wayne State University College of Nursing 6th Annual Summer Research Conference, Detroit, MI.

King, I. M. (1991). Nursing theory 25 years later. *Nursing Science Quarterly, 4*(3), 94-95.

King, I. M. (1992). King's theory of goal attainment. *Nursing Science Quarterly, 5*(1), 19-26.

King, I. M. (1993, June). *King's conceptual system and theory of goal attainment.* Paper presented at the meeting of Sigma Theta Tau International Sixth International Nursing Research Congress, Madrid, Spain.

Lazarus, R. S., & Folkman, S. (1984). *Stress, appraisal, and coping.* New York: Springer.

Magan, S. J. (1987). A critique of King's theory. In Parse, R. R. (Ed.), *Nursing science major paradigms, theories, and critiques.* Philadephia: W. B. Saunders.

Meleis, A. (1991). *Theoretical nursing: Developments and progress* (2nd ed.). Philadelphia: J. B. Lippincott.

Norris, D. M., & Hoyer, P. J. (1993). Dynamism in practice: Parenting within King's framework. *Nursing Science Quarterly, 6*(2), 79-85.

CHAPTER 6

Levine's Conservation Model in Nursing Practice

Karen Moore Schaefer
This chapter is dedicated to the memory of Myra E. Levine.

"Nursing is a profession as well as an academic discipline, always practiced and studied in concert with all of the disciplines that together form the health sciences. . . . Scientific knowledge from many contributing disciplines is, in fact, connected to nursing, as an adjunct to the knowledge that nursing claims for its own." (Levine, 1988)

HISTORY AND BACKGROUND

The conservation model was originally developed as an organizing framework for teaching undergraduate nursing students (Levine, 1973a). Levine's book made a significant contribution to the "whys" of nursing actions. Levine was intent on not simply teaching the skill of nursing but also providing a rationale for the behaviors. She has shown a high regard for the integration of the adjunctive sciences to develop a theoretical basis of nursing, has been a clear voice for the development of the discipline, and continues to call attention to the rhetoric of nursing theory (Levine, 1988, 1989b, 1989c, 1994, 1995).

The universality of the conservation model is supported by its use with a variety of patients of varied ages in a wide range of settings. This model has been successfully used in critical care (Brunner, 1985; Langer, 1990; Litrell & Schumann, 1989; Lynn-McHale & Smith, 1991; Taylor, 1989; Tribotti, 1990), acute care (Foreman, 1991; Molchany, 1992; Schaefer, 1991a), and long-term care (Cox, 1991). The conservation model has also been used with the neonate (Tribotti, 1990), infant (Newport, 1984; Savage & Culbert, 1989), young child (Dever, 1991), pregnant woman

(Roberts, Fleming, & Yeates-Giese, 1991), young adult (Pasco & Halupa, 1991), and elderly (Cox, 1991; Foreman, 1991; Hirschfeld, 1976). It has been successfully used in the community (Pond, 1991), emergency room (Pond & Taney, 1991), extended care facility (Cox, 1991), critical care unit (Brunner, 1985; Molchany, 1992), primary care clinic (Schaefer & Pond, 1994), and operating room (Crawford-Gamble, 1986). The model has been used as a framework for wound care (Cooper, 1990), care of intravenous sites (Dibble, Bostrom-Ezrati & Ruzzuto, 1991), and for patients undergoing treatment for cancer (O'Laughlin, 1986; Webb, 1993). Discussion about its use with the frail elderly is underway (M. Happ, personal communication, January 31, 1995) and consideration is being given to its application in administration (R. A. Cox, personal communication, February 21, 1995). Because of wider use of the conservation model in hospitals and communities, nurse educators are bringing the model into undergraduate and graduate education (Grindley & Paradowski, 1991; Schaefer, 1991b).

OVERVIEW OF LEVINE'S CONSERVATION MODEL

According to Levine (1973a), "nursing is human interaction" (p. 1). "The nurse enters into a partnership of human experience where sharing moments in time—some trivial, some dramatic— leaves its mark forever on each patient" (Levine, 1977, p. 845). As a human science, the profession of nursing integrates the adjunctive sciences (e.g., chemistry, biology, anatomy and physiology, psychology, sociology, anthropology, philosophy, medicine) to develop the practice of nursing.

There are three major concepts that form the basis of the model and its assumptions: conservation, adaptation, and wholeness. *Conservation* is natural law that is fundamental to many basic sciences.

Levine (1973a) explains that individuals are continuously defending their wholeness. Conservation is the *keeping together* of the life system. To *keep together* means to maintain a proper balance between active nursing interventions coupled with patient participation, on the one hand, and the safe limits of the patient's ability to participate on the other. Individuals defend that system in constant interaction with their environment, choosing the most economical, frugal, energy-sparing options available to safeguard their integrity. Energy source cannot be directly observed but the consequences (clinical manifestations) of its exchange are predictable, manageable, and recognizable (Levine, 1991). Conservation is about achieving a balance of energy supply and demand that is within the unique biological realities of the individual.

Adaptation is the ongoing process of change whereby the individuals retain their integrity within the realities of their environment (Levine, 1989a). Change is the life process and adaptation is the method of change. The achievement of adaptation is "the frugal, economic, contained, and controlled use of environmental resources by the individual in his or her best interest" (Levine, 1991, p. 5). Every individual possesses a range of adaptive responses that is unique to that individual. These ranges may vary as one ages or is challenged by illness. This trend is evidenced as the hypoxic drive provides the stimulus for breathing in individuals with chronic obstructive pulmonary disease.

Adaptation is characterized by history, specificity, and redundancy. Adaptations are grounded in history and await the challenges to which they respond (Levine, 1995). The severity of individual responses and their adaptive patterns will vary based on the specific genetic structure and the influence of social, cultural, and experiential factors.

Redundancy represents the fail-safe anatomical, physiological, and psychological options available to the individual to ensure continued adaptation (Levine, 1991). "Achieving health is predicated on the deliberate selection of redundant options" (p. 6). Survival depends on these redundant options, which are challenged and often limited by illness, disease, and aging.

Wholeness exists when the interactions or constant adaptations to the environment permit the assurance of integrity (Levine, 1991). Nurses promote wholeness through the use of the conservation principles. Their recognition of an open, fluid, constantly changing interaction between the individual and the environment is the basis for holistic thought, viewing the individual as whole. Wholeness is health; health is integrity. Health is a pattern of adaptive change, the goal of which is well-being.

The conservation model includes the metaparadigm concepts of person, nursing, health, and environment, which Levine (1988) calls *commonplaces of the discipline* in that they are necessary for any description of nursing. The person is a holistic being who is sentient, thinking, future oriented, and past aware. The wholeness (integrity) of the individual demands that the "isolated aspects . . . can have meaning outside of the context within which the individual experiences his or her life" (Levine, 1973a, pp. 325-326). Persons are in constant interaction with the environment, responding to change in an orderly, sequential pattern. They are thus adapting, and they adapt to forces that shape and reshape the essence of the person. According to Levine (1973a), the person can be defined as an individual, an individual in a group (family), or an individual in a community (Pond, 1991).

The environment completes the wholeness of the person. Each individual is viewed as having his/her own internal and external environments. The internal environment combines the physiological and pathophysiological aspects of the patient. The internal environment is constantly challenged by changes in the external environment.

The external environment includes those factors that impinge on and challenge the individual. Acknowledging the complexity of the environment, Levine (1973a) adopted the three levels of environment identified by Bates (1967). The *perceptual environment* includes aspects of the world that individuals are able to intercept or interpret through the senses. The *operational environment* includes elements that may physically affect individuals but are not directly perceived by them such as radiation and micro-organisms. The *conceptual environment* includes the cultural patterns characterized by spiritual existence and mediated by symbols of language, thought, and history. This includes factors that affect behavior such as values and beliefs.

Health and disease are patterns of adaptive change, one of the goals of which is well-being (Levine, 1971b). Health from a social perspective is defined as, "Do I continue to function in a reasonably normal fashion?" (Levine, 1984). Health (wholeness) is implied as the unity and integrity of the individual. Health (wholeness) is the goal of nursing.

Illness is described as adaptation to noxious environmental forces. "Disease represents the individual's effort to protect self-integrity, such as the inflammatory system's response to injury" (Levine, 1971a, p. 257). Disease is unregulated and undisciplined change and must be stopped or death will ensue (Levine, 1973a).

Nursing involves engaging in "human interaction" (Levine, 1973a, p. 1). The individual seeks nursing care when he/she is no longer able to adapt. The goal of nursing is to promote adaptation and maintain wholeness. This goal is accomplished through the conservation of energy and structural, personal, and social integrity.

Energy conservation depends on the free energy exchange with the environment so that living systems can constantly replenish their energy supply (Levine, 1991). Conservation of energy is integral to the individual's range of adaptive responses. The conservation of structural integrity depends on an intact defense system that supports repair and healing and that is responsive to the challenges from the internal and external environments.

The conservation of personal integrity recognizes the individual who establishes his/her wholeness in response to the environment. It acknowledges that individuals strive for recognition, respect, self-awareness, human-ness, selfhood, and self-determination.

Conservation of social integrity recognizes that individuals function in a society that helps to establish the boundaries of the self. It acknowledges that individuals are valued for their individuality but also have the need to belong to a family, community, religious group, ethnic identity, political system, and nation (Levine, 1973a). "Conservation of integrity is essential to assuring wholeness and providing the strength needed to confront illness and disability" (Levine, 1991, p. 3).

Levine (1973a) makes explicit the importance of understanding the medical plan of care and the results of diagnostic studies to an accurate understanding of patient problems. To this understanding the nurse brings knowledge of nursing science, a careful history of the patient's illness, the patient's perception of the current predicament, information gained from family and friends, and acute observation of the patient and his/her interactions with others (Levine, 1966a). This integrated approach to patient-centered care provides the basis for collaborative care and the establishment of partnerships in the delivery of comprehensive care. Treatment focuses on the management of the organismic responses to the illness.

Organismic responses include flight/fight response, immune system response, stress response, and perceptual awareness. The flight/fight response is the most primitive. The inflammatory/immune response provides for structural continuity and promotion of healing. The stress response is recorded over time and is influenced by the accumulated experience of the individual. Prolonged stress can lead to damage to the systems. The perceptual response involves the gathering of information from the environment and converting it to a meaningful experience. These four responses work together to protect the individual's integrity and are essential components of the individual's whole response.

The goal of nursing care is to promote adaptation and well-being. Because adaptation is predicated on redundant options and rooted in history and specificity, therapeutic interventions will vary based on the unique nature of each person's response.

THEORIES FOR PRACTICE

The model provides the basis for two theories for practice: the theory of therapeutic intention and the theory of redundancy. In developing the theory of therapeutic intention, Levine (as cited in Fawcett, 1995) was "seeking a way of organizing nursing interventions out of the biological realities which the nurse had to confront" (p. 198). Therapeutic regimens should support the following goals (Fawcett, 1995):

1. Facilitate integrated healing and optimal restoration of structure and function through natural response to disease
2. Provide support for a failing autoregulatory portion of the integrated system (medical/surgical treatments)
3. Restore individual integrity and well-being
4. Provide supportive measures to ensure comfort and promote human concern when therapeutic measures are not possible
5. Balance a toxic risk against the threat of disease
6. Manipulate diet and activity to correct metabolic imbalances and to stimulate physiological processes
7. Reinforce or antagonize usual response to create a therapeutic change

Levine (as cited in Fawcett, 1995) proposed that the theory of redundancy, seemingly grounded in adaptation, "redefines almost everything that has to do with human life" (p. 199). Redundancy seems to be predicated on the ability of the individual to "monitor its own behavior by conserving the use of resources required to define their unique identity (Levine, 1991, p. 4). Inherent in this ability to select from the environment is the availability of options from which choices can be made.

CRITICAL THINKING IN NURSING PRACTICE WITH LEVINE'S MODEL

Levine (1973a, 1973b) proposes that nurses use their scientific and creative abilities to provide nursing care to the patient. The nursing process incorporates these abilities, enhancing the nurse's ability to think critically about the patient's predicament. See Table 6-1 for Levine's nursing process using critical thinking.

TABLE 6-1   Levine's Nursing Process Using Critical Thinking

Process	Decision Making
ASSESSMENT	
Collection of provocative facts through interview and observation of challenges to environments, with consideration of conservation principles	Nurse observes patient for organismic responses to illness, reads medical reports, evaluates results of diagnostic studies, and talks with patient about his/her needs for assistance. Nurse assesses for challenges to both internal and external environments of patient. Guided by conservation principles, nurse assesses for additional challenges in environments. Nurse assesses for challenges that interfere with:*
1. Energy conservation	1. Balance of energy supply and demand.
2. Structural integrity	2. Body's defense system.
3. Personal integrity	3. Person's sense of self-worth and personhood.
4. Social integrity	4. Person's ability to participate in social system. These data are provocative facts.
JUDGMENT—TROPHICOGNOSIS†	
Nursing diagnosis—gives the provocative facts meaning	Provocative facts are arranged in a way that they provide meaning to patient's predicament. A judgment is made about patient's needs for assistance. This judgment is the trophicognosis.†

*Although use of the conservation principles to guide the assessment of challenges in the environments was not part of the original model, it helps the novice nurse, in particular, to organize the provocative facts in a manner that directs the hypotheses. For the experienced nurse, this is integrated into the assessment of the environments as in nursing care of Alice (see text).
†*Trophicognosis* is a nursing care judgment arrived at through the use of the scientific process (Levine, 1966b). The scientific process is used to make observations and select relevant data to form hypothetical statements about the patient's predicaments (Schaefer, 1991a).

TABLE 6-1   Levine's Nursing Process Using Critical Thinking—cont'd

Process	Decision Making
HYPOTHESES	
Direct the nursing interventions with the goal of maintaining wholeness and promoting adaptation	Based on nurse's judgment, nurse seeks validation with patient about problem. Nurse then proposes hypotheses about problem and its solution. This becomes the plan of care.
INTERVENTIONS	
Tests hypothesis	Nurse uses hypothesis to direct care. In essence, the nurse tests proposed hypotheses. Interventions are designed based on conservation principles: conservation of energy, structural integrity, personal integrity, and social integrity. The expectation is that this approach will maintain wholeness and promote adaptation.
EVALUATION	
Observation of organismic response to interventions	The outcome of hypothesis testing is evaluated by assessing for organismic response that means the hypothesis was supported or not supported. Consequences of care are either therapeutic or supportive: therapeutic improves one's sense of well-being; supportive provides comfort when downward course of illness cannot be influenced. If hypothesis is not supported, plan is revised and new hypothesis is proposed.

CASE HISTORY OF DEBBIE

Debbie is a 29-year-old woman who was recently admitted to the oncology nursing unit for evaluation after sensing pelvic "fullness" and noticing a watery, foul-smelling vaginal discharge. A Papanicolaou smear revealed a class V cervical cancer. She was found to have a stage II squamous cell carcinoma of the cervix and underwent a radical hysterectomy with bilateral salpingooophorectomy.

Her past health history revealed that physical examinations had been infrequent. She also reported that she had not performed breast self-examination. She is 5 feet 4 inches tall and weighs 89 pounds. Her usual weight is about 110 pounds. She has smoked approximately two packs of cigarettes a day for the past 16 years. She is gravida 2, para 2. Her first pregnancy was at age 16, and her second was at age 18. Since that time she has taken oral contraceptives on a regular basis.

Debbie completed the eighth grade. She is married and lives with her husband and two children in her mother's home, which she describes as less than sanitary. Her husband is unemployed. She describes him as emotionally distant and abusive at times.

She has done well following surgery except for being unable to completely empty her urinary bladder. She is having continued postoperative pain and nausea. It will be necessary for her to perform intermittent self-catheterization at home. Her medications are (1) an antibiotic, (2) an analgesic as needed for pain, and (3) an antiemetic as needed for nausea. In addition, she will be receiving radiation therapy on an outpatient basis.

Debbie is extremely tearful. She expresses great concern over her future and the future of her two children. She believes that this illness is a punishment for her past life.

NURSING CARE OF DEBBIE WITH LEVINE'S MODEL

Debbie is very concerned about her future and the future of her children. Debbie requires nursing care because of the environmental challenges that have threatened her integrity and interfered with her ability to adapt. The nurse assesses for the challenges to her internal and external environments.

Challenges to Debbie's Internal Environment

Challenges that reduce Debbie's energy resources include weight loss of 20 pounds and smoking. She has had radical surgery, which challenges her structural integrity. The resulting loss of reproductive ability poses a challenge to her personal integrity. Subsequent to the surgery she is having difficulty completely emptying her bladder. She smokes and has taken oral contraceptives on a regular basis. The results of diagnostic studies and vital signs would provide additional indices about the challenges to her internal environment.

Challenges to Debbie's External Environment

Debbie's husband is emotionally distant and at times abusive. Given these facts, the nurse would investigate available patient records for any indication (bruises, burns, broken bones, chronic pain) that the abuse has been the reason for other healthcare visits.

She is living in a home that she describes as "less than sanitary." She is concerned about her future and the future of her two children.

Assessment

Energy conservation. Challenges that result in an energy drain of Debbie's resources include recent weight loss, nausea, pain, and smoking. She has pain even though she has pain medication ordered. She is concerned about the care of her two children.

Structural integrity. Debbie's structural integrity is threatened by a surgical procedure with the potential for skin breakdown and infection. She is currently receiving an antibiotic prophylactically to prevent infection of the surgical wound. In addition, she is having difficulty emptying her bladder. Risk assessment includes oral contraceptive administration, smoking, early childbirth, and her recent diagnosis of cancer. On discharge she will undergo radiation therapy. Radiation therapy poses additional challenges of skin breakdown, destruction of normal cells, pain, potential nausea, and hair loss in the irradiated area.

Personal integrity. Debbie feels as though her illness is a punishment for past behaviors. The surgery and the consequences of the surgical technique may further jeopardize her sense of self-worth. Debbie is only 29 years old and she could have had more children were it not for this surgery. The impact of not being able to give birth to more children could be devastating. Further, the impact of this situation on the family must be considered. Debbie identifies her husband as being emotionally distant and acknowledges that he may not be capable of providing her with emotional support.

Social integrity. Debbie will experience premature menopause and all the emotional and physical effects of the experience. Many young women her age have infants and menstrual cycles; she will not. Her own and her children's concern about whether she will be there to raise them may cause considerable anxiety and fear about the future. Debbie's relationship with her husband may experience added strain. The emotional impact of the surgery on him and his potential for abusive behavior must be evaluated.

Judgments
The following trophicognoses (diagnoses) are identified for Debbie:
1. Inadequate nutritional status
2. Pain
3. Engaging in risky behavior
4. Potential for wound and bladder infection
5. Need to learn self-catheterization
6. Preparation for radiation therapy
7. Decreased self-worth, feeling guilty
8. Potential for abuse

9. Premature menopause
10. Concern for her children's future

Hypotheses

Using the conservation model, the nurse proposes hypotheses about Debbie's needs to develop a plan of care with her. Some of the hypotheses might include:

1. Providing Debbie with a nutritional consultation will assist her with finding foods that she can tolerate and foods that will provide her with the energy she needs for strength and healing.
2. Careful use of food and medicine for nausea will improve her tolerance for food.
3. Adequate teaching and return demonstration of urinary self-catheterization will reduce the potential for infection.
4. Observation and cleansing of the surgical wound will reduce the chance for infection.
5. Preparation for radiation treatment that includes the expected effects and ways to reduce the effects will promote structural integrity (maintain skin integrity) and personal integrity (provide the patient with control if she desires some control).
6. Encouraging Debbie to talk about what having a hysterectomy means to her, her concerns, and her fears will help her to resolve fears, defuse myths associated with loss of femininity, and prepare her for some of the emotional/physical effects including premature menopause.
7. Providing Debbie with a visiting nurse follow-up visit (post-discharge visit) will provide her with emotional (sharing) and physical support (self-catheterization reinforcement).
8. Teaching her about her discharge medications will maximize their effect (pain relief) and reduce the risk of potential side effects.
9. Teaching alternate approaches for pain management (relaxation) will increase the effects of the pain medication.
10. Providing information about risky behaviors that includes ways to reduce those behaviors will give Debbie control over her health and reduce or control risky behaviors.
11. Providing her with time to talk about why she thinks her diagnosis is punishment for past behavior will help her to understand that she did not cause her illness and subsequently will improve her sense of self-worth.

Nursing Interventions

When providing care to Debbie, the nurse uses the conservation principles to maintain wholeness and promote adaptation.

Energy conservation. A nutritional consultation will assist Debbie in identifying foods that will reduce nausea, improve caloric intake, and maintain the required intake for her size. If nausea continues, careful administration of the medication before eating may help to reduce associated nausea. The frequency and intensity of the pain can be controlled by identifying those activities that aggravate the pain and by offering the medication or other pain management interventions to reduce the pain. Because patients frequently experience fatigue after a total hysterectomy and as a result of the radiation treatment, Debbie will be prepared for normal fatigue and how to balance her activity and rest periods. Rest will become very important while the body is healing.

Structural integrity. Debbie's wound will be assessed for signs of healing. The antibiotic will be administered as ordered with instructions on how she is to take it once she returns home. The nurse will stress the importance of completing the prescriptions as ordered.

Debbie will be taught self-catheterization. Return demonstrations will improve her confidence in performing the task.

Before discharge Debbie will be prepared for radiation treatments on an outpatient basis. The following points should be stressed: the importance of laboratory work to monitor the body's response to the therapy, the importance of skin protection to reduce skin irritation associated with the radiation, and the avoidance of situations that support infection (child with a cold) because of the body's decreased ability to fight infection.

Personal integrity. Debbie will be encouraged to talk about having her uterus removed because of cancer. If she chooses not to discuss how she feels, the nurse will respect her privacy.

Because Debbie feels that her illness is punishment for her past behavior, Debbie needs to be reassured. If appropriate, a referral to a mental health clinical nurse specialist should be made.

Social integrity. The nurse will also assess the potential for abuse from Debbie's husband and family needs for support.

Organismic Responses

In response to the interventions, the nurse would observe for the following possible organismic responses:

1. Abdominal wound healing
2. Clean urinary self-catheterization
3. Dialogue about how Debbie feels about the hysterectomy and cancer
4. Improved appetite and weight gain
5. Recognition that her past behavior did not cause the disease

6. Restful sleep and increased energy level
7. Controlled pain
8. Husband and children are providing assistance within their capabilities

ASE HISTORY OF ALICE

Alice was diagnosed with fibromyalgia (FM) in 1988. At the time of the assessment she was 44 years old, married, and without children. She worked as a secretary for temporary services requiring computer skills. She had quit her full-time job because of the extreme stress of the environment and the overtime hours required. I met her when she had inquired about a study to examine the health patterns of women with FM. She described herself as desperate for anything that would help her. I clarified for her that the study was not meant to help her but to describe the patterns of health in women with the disorder. With her permission, her story is used as an exemplar for the use of Levine's conservation model.

At the time of assessment, Alice had been missing a lot of work because of the amount of pain and fatigue she was experiencing when she got up in the morning. Her pain was severe enough that she was unable to lift a cup of coffee. At times she had difficulty cleaning herself after bowel movements because of the pain in her arm when she extended it backward. Sometimes her pain and fatigue were so severe that she had to cancel social engagements. This situation often resulted in her feeling sorry for herself and bouts of crying. Severe headaches were of particular concern for her. She reported that her libido was significantly decreased. She said her husband told her that she has a split personality: when she is not tired, she is fine; when she is getting tired, she verbally attacks him and is mean. Her husband tried to be understanding, but his patience was wearing thin.

She was under the care of a physician who had prescribed an antidepressant. She chose not to take any medication except an anti-inflammatory medication for menstrual cramps. She was particularly adverse to taking the antidepressant because she knew it was an antidepressant. Her physician had ruled out all other possible sources of pain through his diagnostic workup and that of a consulting neurologist. She was searching for help and had thought about going to support group meetings but had not done so at the time of assessment. She was continuously trying to determine what she did or ate that might cause her pain and fatigue so that she might change patterns even during a single day. She had learned that pacing herself when she had a lot to do helped to reduce the intensity of the pain experience. Massage at times temporarily reduced the achiness and pain. She observed that damp rainy weather made her feel worse. She agreed to keep a daily diary to help identify her patterns of health and illness. It was hoped that this would provide her with information about her predicament and give her some control over her health.

NURSING CARE OF ALICE WITH LEVINE'S MODEL

Fibromyalgia (FM) is a chronic painful muscle disorder that is most commonly first diagnosed in women between the ages of 20 and 45 years

(Rothchild, 1991). Most diagnostic studies are normal, yet the individuals feel terrible. The symptoms generally mimic the flu with muscle aches and pains, stiffness, nausea, and fatigue (Boissevain & McCain, 1991).

According to Levine (1971a), the focus of nursing care is the maintenance of wholeness (integrity, oneness) and the promotion of adaptation. Alice was very open to discussion about what she might be able to do for herself. She was desperate and frustrated with the notion that nothing seemed to be helping her.

Continuous pain and fatigue were getting her down. She continued to see her physician, who ordered additional testing to ensure that nothing new was causing the pain. In the interim she was seeking some relief. Levine's conservation model directs the nurse to involve the patients in decisions about their care.

As the nurse entered into a relationship with Alice, she encouraged her to explain her predicament. Attention to the environmental factors and the integrities help nurses to ensure that the patient's sense of oneness is maintained even during an initial encounter. Patients often doubt their integrity and feel, like Alice, that they no longer have control over their lives, they are not taken seriously, and their concerns are not perceived as valid (Schaefer, 1995).

Challenges to Alice's Internal Environment

Assessment revealed that Alice had "been treating pains for years." All the diagnostic tests were normal. She reported a history of difficult menstrual periods, premenstrual syndrome (PMS), and migraine headaches. All the physiological and pathophysiological aspects of her internal environment were found to be normal.

Challenges to Alice's External Environment

Alice noticed that she experienced migraine headaches after she ate Italian food and concluded that she might be allergic to the sauce. She claimed she felt better since she began being more careful, thus supporting Levine's notion that a person seeks, selects, and tests information from the environment in the context of his/her definition of self, thus defending his/her safety, identity, and purpose (1991).

Adaptation to the conceptual environment is sometimes threatened by the response that implies that the complaints associated with the illness are not valid. Alice was fortunate that her physicians acknowledged her pain; however, family members had a difficult time believing that there really was something wrong. Socially, she felt as though people thought she was malingering, and she felt sorry for herself when she could not keep her social engagements.

Judgment (Trophicognosis)

Alice was diagnosed with FM, a chronic illness about which little is known. The major problems are fatigue and pain, which have threatened her ability to adapt and maintain wholeness. Considering the conservation principles, the nurse tried to help her adapt in a positive manner and to help her return to a level of perceived wholeness.

Hypotheses

1. Encouraging the combined use of pharmacological and non-pharmacological sleep interventions (relaxation, hot showers) will improve the subjective quality of Alice's sleep and improve her energy level.
2. Loss of weight will help reduce Alice's aches and pains.
3. Encouraging Alice to keep a diary of her symptoms and the internal and external environmental challenges to her integrity will improve Alice's understanding of her unique patterns of FM.
4. Adequate teaching about the medications Alice can take for FM will help her make a decision about the use of pharmacological interventions.
5. Encouraging Alice to communicate openly and honestly will help reduce the anger she feels.
6. When Alice feels physically better, she will feel better about herself and will be able to engage in social activities.

Nursing Interventions

Energy conservation. Both emotional stress and managing multiple responsibilities at work and home was an energy drain for Alice. She elected to work part-time rather than stay in an environment that seemed unhealthy for her.

Alice reported in her diary that she frequently had difficulty getting a good night's sleep. She believed that the more restless her night, the more pain she experienced in the morning. Her diary supported this claim. Sleep improved slightly when she used her relaxation tapes to fall asleep. The nurse suggested that her sleep may be improved by taking a warm bath before bedtime, drinking warm milk at bedtime, and avoiding heavy foods 3 to 4 hours before bedtime. She was encouraged to establish a bedtime routine that she practiced on a daily basis. The notion of routine is critical to these interventions.

When discussing possible ways to improve Alice's sleep, the nurse reviewed the drugs Alice was taking and the possible effects. It was at this time that Alice indicated that she had a prescription for an antidepressant but she chose not to take it. The nurse informed Alice that the drug is frequently helpful in reducing the severity and frequency of pain but that it may take up to 3 weeks for the benefits to be noticed. She also told her that women have stopped taking the drug because of the inability to tolerate the side effects. She reviewed the effects of dry mouth, fast pulse, and constipation, noting that eating a diet with grains and vegetables and drinking 10 glasses of water a day reduces these side effects. Alice tried taking the medicine but did so only sporadically. She found that if she took the drug every night she felt much better and had a greater amount of energy. She was subsequently able to plan social outings without the constant fear that she would have to cancel her plans because of the pain and fatigue.

Alice had identified the importance of pacing activities when she had a lot to do. Planning for additional sleep needs was an extension of her established pattern of behavior. During times of stress (e.g., deadlines at work, illness, menstrual periods), she would plan to get extra sleep at night or find a time when she could nap in the afternoon. If sleep is not possible, rest accompanied by relaxation, such as slow rhythmic breathing and imagery, has the potential to replenish energy needs.

Alice was about 10 pounds overweight. She agreed to try to slowly lose some of the weight. Her physician believed that with weight reduction the strain on her back would decrease and would control her aches and pains.

Alice noted that she thought foods such as tomatoes or spices precipitated her headaches. She was encouraged to keep a record of the food she ate and the pattern of symptoms she experienced.

A review of her diary, her reported experiences, and the results of cross-correlation analysis revealed that weather changes lagged the pain and fatigue by up to 2 days. This helped her to realize that some of the pain and fatigue was temporary and would decrease once the weather actually changed. This recognition helped her deal with the discomfort in a more positive way if only to simply get more rest when challenged by external environmental factors.

Structural integrity. Alice understood that, because of the uncertainty about the symptoms, other illness must be "ruled out" to ensure that appropriate interventions were ordered. Because Alice was taking antidepressants, she needed to know about the possibility of weight gain, dry membranes, and constipation. Eating complex carbohydrates can help reduce the hunger associated with the increased serotonin levels. Drinking more water and eating a balanced diet may help reduce the dryness and constipation. Heart rate changes are associated with some antidepressants and should be reported to the physician or nurse practitioner. She was also reassured that alternative medications are available if she is unable to tolerate the prescribed drug. Because she expressed an interest in homeopathy, she was warned that herbs and other over-the-counter remedies can be equally harmful and she should not take any of these homeopathic treatments without supervision.

Alice was encouraged to continue taking hot showers in the morning and listening to her tapes at night. Because she admitted to having a few alcoholic drinks before bed, she was encouraged to not drink more than two and to avoid drinking for 3 hours before bedtime.

Personal integrity. Regaining a sense of selfhood for Alice meant being able to do things around the house and to enjoy social events with her husband and family. She expressed satisfaction with the fact that she "seemed to be getting better" and could do most of the things she hoped to be able to do.

Social integrity. It was suggested to Alice that attending a support group might help. Alice said the support groups made her feel excited, she finally found people who have the same problem she does, she has learned a lot about her illness, she likes interacting with the other members, and she feels good when she attends the meetings. Alice is a very outgoing person, and with her pain under control she has been able to reach out to other people at the support groups.

It is important to encourage the patient to communicate openly and honestly. Alice felt that her husband did not really understand her illness; he simply tolerated it. Although this made her angry, it also gave her cause for concern that their marriage was suffering. Alice made the choice to attend support groups and when she shared her positive experience with her husband, she had her first "emotional feeling" talk with him in years. She felt extremely good about this.

Organismic Responses

Success of the interventions is measured through the observation of organismic responses. Responses observed in Alice included (1) reduction in reported pain or need for pain control, (2) reported improved quality of sleep, (3) reported improved ability to anticipate and plan for exacerbations, (4) better understanding of illness, (5) comfort in sharing of stories, (6) reduction in stress, (7) reported improved quality of life, (8) better communication with husband, (9) increased energy, and (10) satisfaction because she was feeling better.

CRITICAL THINKING EXERCISES

1. Select and read a pathography (autobiography or biography involving a story about illness) of interest to you in your area of clinical practice (e.g., *The Alchemy of Illness;* Duff, 1993). Use Levine's conservation model to evaluate the health and healthcare of the individual in the story. Consider the medical plan of care, environmental challenges, and organismic responses. Evaluate the use of the model relative to the identification of the nursing care needs of the patient and the potential use of the model in promoting adaptation and maintaining wholeness. Explore how the patient defines adaptation and wholeness. What questions would be asked to gather the information found in the book? Compare these questions to the questions that would be asked if you were using Levine's conservation model. Make a judgment about the value of the model with attention to its strengths and weaknesses.

2. Write a story about when you were ill or when a family member or friend was ill. Given the nature of the illness, what was needed for you or the friend/family member to feel well? How would you help them get to that point? What were the actual outcomes and how would the use of the conservation model change or support those outcomes?

3. List the assumptions on which Levine's conservation model is based. Determine if the assumptions are or are not consistent with your beliefs. Identify the knowledge that supports these assumptions. Determine how you could support or refute their validity (truthfulness).

4. Consider and write about a nursing situation that you have recently encountered. Use this situation to determine the kind of knowledge needed to provide nursing care. Distinguish between that which is nursing knowledge and that which is knowledge from the adjunctive disciplines. Determine how adjunctive knowledge becomes nursing knowledge in this situation. What knowledge is missing? What other information is needed?

References

Bates, M. (1967). A naturalist at large. *Natural History, 76*(6), 8-16.

Boissevain, M. D., & McCain, G. A. (1991). Toward an integrated understanding of fibromyalgia syndrome: II. Psychological and phenomenological aspects. *Pain, 45,* 239-248.

Brunner, M. (1985). A conceptual approach to critical care nursing using Levine's model. *Focus on Critical Care, 12*(2), 39-44.

Cooper, D. H. (1990). Optimizing wound healing: A practice within nursing domains. *Nursing Clinics of North America, 25*(1), 165-180.

Cox, R. A., Sr. (1991). A tradition of caring: Use of Levine's model in long-term care. In K. M. Schaefer & J. B. Pond (Eds.), *The conservation model: A framework for nursing practice* (pp. 179-197). Philadelphia: F. A. Davis.

Crawford-Gamble, P. E. (1986). An application of Levine's conceptual model. *Perioperative Nursing Quarterly, 2*(1), 64-70.

Dever, M. (1991). Care of children. In K. M. Schaefer & J. B. Pond (Eds.), *The conservation model: A framework for nursing practice* (pp. 71-82). Philadelphia: F. A. Davis.

Dibble, S. L., Bostrom-Ezrati, J., & Ruzzuto, C. (1991). Clinical predictors of intravenous site symptoms. *Research in Nursing & Health, 14,* 413-420.

Duff, K. (1993). *The alchemy of illness.* New York: Pantheon Books.

Fawcett, J. (1995). *Conceptual models of nursing* (3rd ed.). Philadelphia: F. A. Davis.

Foreman, M. D. (1991). Conserving cognitive integrity of the hospitalized elderly. In K. M. Schaefer & J. B. Pond (Eds.), *The conservation model: A framework for nursing practice* (pp. 133-150). Philadelphia: F. A. Davis.

Grindley, J., & Paradowski, M. B. (1991). Developing an undergraduate program using Levine's model. In K. M. Schaefer & J. B. Pond (Eds.), *The conservation model: A framework for nursing practice* (pp. 199-208). Philadelphia: F. A. Davis.

Hirschfeld, M. H. (1976). The cognitively impaired older adult. *American Journal of Nursing, 76,* 1981-1984.

Langer, V. S. (1990). Minimal handling protocol for the intensive care nursery. *Neonatal Network, 9*(3), 23-27.

Levine, M. E. (1966a). Adaptation and assessment: A rationale for nursing intervention. *American Journal of Nursing, 66,* 2450-2453.

Levine, M. E. (1966b). Trophicognosis: An alternative to nursing diagnosis. In *American Nurses' Association Regional Clinical Conference* (vol. 2, pp. 55-70). New York: American Nurses Association.

Levine, M. E. (1971a). Holistic nursing. *Nursing Clinics of North America, 6*(2), 253-263.

Levine, M. E. (1971b). *Renewal for nursing.* Philadelphia: F. A. Davis.

Levine, M. E. (1973a). *Introduction to clinical nursing* (2nd ed.). Philadelphia: F. A. Davis.

Levine, M. E. (1973b). On creativity in nursing. *Image, 3*(3), 15-19.

Levine, M. E. (1977). Nursing ethics and the ethical nurse. *American Journal of Nursing, 77*(5), 845-849.

Levine, M. E. (1984, August). *Myra Levine.* Paper presented at the Nurse Theorist Conference, Edmonton, Alberta, Canada. (Cassette recording).

Levine, M. E. (1988). Antecedents from adjunctive disciplines: Creation of nursing theory. *Nursing Science Quarterly, 1*(1), 16-21.

Levine, M. E. (1989a). The conservation model: Twenty years later. In J. P. Riehl-Sisca (Ed.), *Conceptual models for nursing practice* (pp. 325-337), Norwalk, CT: Appleton & Lange.

Levine, M. E. (1989b). Ration or rescue: The elderly in critical care. *Critical Care Nursing, 12*(1), 82-89.

Levine, M. E. (1989c). The ethics of nursing rhetoric. *Image: Journal of Nursing Scholarship, 21*(1), 4-5.

Levine, M. E. (1991). The conservation model: A model for health. In K. M. Schaefer & J. B. Pond (Eds.), *The conservation model: A framework for nursing practice* (pp. 1-11). Philadelphia: F. A. Davis.

Levine, M. E. (1994). Some further thoughts on nursing rhetoric. In J. F. Kikuchi & H. Simmons (Eds.), *Developing a philosophy of nursing* (pp. 104-109). Thousand Oaks, CA: Sage Publications.

Levine, M. E. (1995). The rhetoric of nursing theory. *Image: Journal of Nursing Scholarship, 27*(1), 11-14.

Litrell, K, & Schumann, L. (1989). Promoting sleep for the patient with a myocardial infarction. *Critical Care Nurse, 9*(3), 44-49.

Lynn-McHale, D. J., & Smith, A. (1991). Comprehensive assessment of families of the critically ill. In J. S. Leske (Ed.), *AACN Clinical Issues in Critical Care Nursing* (pp. 195-209). Philadelphia: J. B. Lippincott.

Molchany, C. A. (1992). Ventricular septal and free wall rupture complicating acute MI. *Journal of Cardiovascular Nursing, 6*(4), 38-45.

Newport, M. A. (1984). Conserving thermal energy and social integrity in the newborn. *Western Journal of Nursing Research, 6*(2), 175-197.

O'Laughlin, K. M. (1986). Changes in bladder function in the woman undergoing radical hysterectomy for cervical cancer. *JOGNN, 15*(5), 380-385.

Pasco, A., & Halupa, D. (1991). Chronic pain management. In K. M. Schaefer & J. B. Pond (Eds.), *The conservation model: A framework for practice* (pp. 101-117). Philadelphia: F. A. Davis.

Pond, J. B. (1991). Ambulatory care of the homeless. In K. M. Schaefer & J. B. Pond (Eds.), *The conservation model: A framework for practice* (pp. 167-178). Philadelphia: F. A. Davis.

Pond, J. B., & Taney, S. G. (1991). Emergency care in a large university emergency department. In K. M. Schaefer & J. B. Pond (Eds.), *The conservation model: A framework for practice* (pp. 151-166). Philadelphia: F. A. Davis.

Roberts, J. E., Fleming, N., & Yeates-Giese, D. (1991). Perineal integrity. In K. M. Schaefer & J. B. Pond (Eds.), *The conservation model: A framework for practice* (pp. 61-70). Philadelphia: F. A. Davis.

Rothchild, B. M. (1991). Fibromyalgia: An explanation for the aches and pains of the nineties. *Comprehensive Therapy, 17*(6), 9-14.

Savage, T. A., & Culbert, C. (1989). Early intervention: The unique role of nursing. *Journal of Pediatric Nursing, 4*(5), 339-345.

Schaefer, K. (1991a). Care of the patient with congestive heart failure. In K. M. Schaefer & J. B. Pond (Eds.), *The conservation model: A framework for practice* (pp. 119-132). Philadelphia: F. A. Davis.

Schaefer, K. (1991b). Developing a graduate program in nursing: Integrating Levine's philosophy. In K. M. Schaefer & J. B. Pond (Eds.), *The conservation model: A framework for practice* (pp. 209-218). Philadelphia: F. A. Davis.

Schaefer, K. M. (1995). Struggling to maintain balance: A study of women with fibromyalgia. *Journal of Advanced Nursing, 21,* 95-102.

Schaefer, K. M., & Pond, J. B. (1994). Levine's conservation model as a guide to nursing practice. *Nursing Science Quarterly, 7*(2), 53-54.

Taylor, J. W. (1989). Levine's conservation principles. Using the model for nursing diagnosis in a neurological setting. In J. P. Riehl-Sisca (Ed.), *Conceptual models for nursing practice* (3rd ed., pp. 349-358). Norwalk, CT: Appleton & Lange.

Tribotti, S. (1990). Admission to the neonatal intensive care unit: Reducing the risks. *Neonatal Network, 8*(4), 17-22.

Webb, H. (1993). Holistic care following a palliative Hartmann's procedure. *British Journal of Nursing, 2*(2), 128-132.

Neuman's Systems Model in Nursing Practice

Raphella Sohier

"Wholism, implicit in the Neuman systems model, is both a philosophical and a biological concept, implying relationships and processes arising from wholeness, dynamic freedom, and creativity in adjusting to stressors in the internal and external environments. Using a wholistic systems approach to both protect and promote client welfare, nursing action must be skillfully related to the meaningful and dynamic organization of the various parts and subparts of the whole affecting the client. The various interrelationships of the parts and subparts must be appropriately identified before relevant nursing action can be taken." (Neuman, 1995)

HISTORY AND BACKGROUND

Neuman first designed her systems model in the early 1970s as a teaching tool to assist psychiatric/mental health nursing students in their early encounters with clients in community mental health centers. Neuman conceptualizes the "client system" or focus of nursing practice as a person, dyad, family unit, group, population stratum, entire community, or society (Neuman & Young, 1972; Neuman, 1974, 1980, 1982, 1989a, 1989b, 1990, 1995). Literature addressing the application of the Neuman systems model in practice with each of these foci can be found in the major works on Neuman (1990, 1995). The model has been extensively applied in practice and in educational and management settings and has been a focus for research. In the final section of her recent book, Neuman (1995) discusses the trajectory from the past, into the present, and on into the future, detailing the uses of the model in all of these settings (pp. 669-703).

Each client system, whether an individual or an aggregate, is visualized as an open system experiencing stressors that can develop from internal as well as external environments. Neuman (1995) explains that a systems perspective was chosen for her model because it permits "the precise comprehensive analysis of the relations in space and time on which they [the clients] largely depend" (p. 10).

Systems models have two equally important features: structure and process. All systems consist of subsystems. Each subsystem and each system is complete in itself. The sum of the subsystems or parts that comprise the system is said to be "greater than the sum of its parts" (von Bertalanffy, 1968). As open systems, human systems accept input from outside the system, process the input in a phase called *throughput*, and export it in a phase called *output*. Equilibrium or a stable state is the goal of the system. Change (e.g., input, throughput, output) is a feature of the process and the end product (output) is of necessity different from that which is entered into the system (input). Neuman describes people as open systems in constant interaction with the internal and external environments.

The Neuman systems model is health oriented. Neuman (1995) describes health on a continuum from well to ill and speaks of an "optimal state of wellness" as "the best possible state of health for a client system at any given point in time" (p. 32). Equilibrium or a stable state is the healthy state of the system, and disequilibrium is the unhealthy or diseased state of the system. Neuman offers a general proposition that the healthier a system is, the lower the reaction to stress will be, the greater the control over disequilibrium, and the faster a return to stability can be achieved. Prevention of disequilibrium or illness is a central focus and goal; thus Neuman (1995) describes her model as a wellness model.

OVERVIEW OF NEUMAN'S SYSTEMS MODEL

"The intent of the Neuman systems model or conceptual framework is to set forth a structure that depicts the parts and subparts and their interrelationship for the whole of the client as a complete system" (Neuman, 1995, p. 15). Neuman depicts the client system as a person or persons constantly bombarded by environmental stressors (Selye, 1950). Whereas the client system is exposed to stressors from within and without the system, as visualized by Neuman, the client system is also protected by a series of concentric buffers that serve to minimize the impact of stressors and act as safety zones between environments and the central core. The greater the quality of the client system's health, the greater the protection provided by the buffers or safety zones. The central core consists of functions basic or essential to human life. When the client system is in equilibrium (well), all the protective circles are in place. Figure 7-1 provides a visual depiction of Neuman's model.

Beginning at the outside, we encounter the *flexible line of defense* (FLD). This protective mechanism has a great deal of flexibility with an accordian-like effect in the healthy client system. If the client takes appropriate health measures (e.g., eats a healthy diet, gets adequate rest), the client system can tolerate normal life stress and even extraordinary stress for a time. When the system is healthy, the FLD is extended far away from the next buffer called the *normal line of defense* (NLD). As long as stressors are not extreme and the organism continues to live in a healthy manner, the flexibility of this buffer will permit a measure of give-and-take. For example, a busy student who has a part-time job, a full-time school schedule, and shared responsibility for home and children will survive as long as he/she eats properly, exercises, rests appropriately, and gets some recreation. However, if this person ignores body language (tiredness) or body needs (hunger), resistance is weakened and susceptibility to stressors is increased, and very soon he/she will

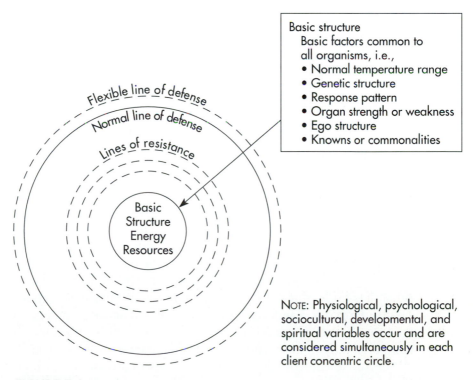

Basic structure
   Basic factors common to
   all organisms, i.e.,
     • Normal temperature range
     • Genetic structure
     • Response pattern
     • Organ strength or weakness
     • Ego structure
     • Knowns or commonalities

Flexible line of defense
Normal line of defense
Lines of resistance

Basic
Structure
Energy
Resources

NOTE: Physiological, psychological, sociocultural, developmental, and spiritual variables occur and are considered simultaneously in each client concentric circle.

FIGURE 7-1

The client system. (From Neuman, B. [1995]. *The Neuman systems model* [3rd ed.]. Norwalk, CT: Appleton & Lange.)

become vulnerable to a common infection such as a cold virus. The FLD will be breached and the normal line of defense, the NLD, will be threatened. In the same fashion, without appropriate action to care for the system, a common cold may become bronchitis or even pneumonia. At that point the NLD has also been breached and the internal buffer, called the *lines of resistance* (LOR) or the life-protecting buffer, is threatened. In that case, if the pneumonia state becomes acute, a life-threatening situation can arise.

When the client system is well, stable, and in equilibrium, the protective mechanisms are all in place. As these mechanisms are breached, the client enters a state of disequilibrium during which nursing interventions are called for. In order to intervene using the Neuman model, the nurse must understand that stressors threatening the integrity of the system may be intrapersonal, interpersonal, or extrapersonal in nature. For example, if the client system is a person with a medical condition, that condition constitutes an *intrapersonal* stressor. If the client system is a family in disequilibrium, the stressor is *interpersonal* in nature. If the client system is a community that has experienced an external threat, the stressor is an *extrapersonal* stressor. Often stressors of all three types are at work simultaneously in the lives of clients.

In order to determine the nature of the stressors affecting clients and to provide direction for the nursing process, the nurse carries out a thorough and "wholistic assessment" (Neuman, 1995, p. 10). The client system is assessed from five perspectives: physiological, psychological, developmental, sociocultural, and spiritual. At first contact with the client, the assessment is carried out in great detail. At later contacts, it may be sufficient to update the original assessment.

Addressing the variables one by one provides the detail essential for an accurate diagnosis and differential diagnoses. In order to maintain the wholistic focus central to Neuman's model, the assessment data relating to the five variables are reintegrated to form a wholistic picture of the client system. Neuman focuses on the client's perspective, which is obtained by addressing several questions to the client regarding the problem that brings him/her to the care provider. The objective results from the nursing assessment are fed back to the client to ensure that the nurse has understood the problem from the client's perspective (Sohier, 1995). Primary diagnosis and differential diagnoses emerge through analysis of the data and are congruent with this subjective-objective comparison. A plan of care is constituted based on these data.

The nurse categorizes the data in terms of stressors and their nature (intrapersonal, interpersonal, or extrapersonal). The data are shared with the client system, individual or aggregate feedback is considered and incorporated in the data, and the client is encouraged to express all opinions regarding the accuracy of the conclusion at this step and throughout the nursing process. When appropriate nursing interventions have been agreed on, the client is encouraged to comment on whether he/she believes the goals can be achieved by this or that method. Sometimes it may be appropriate to contract with the client about how goals are to be achieved and to share responsibility between the client and the provider for meeting them. This feature of caregiver-client cooperation in the application of the Neuman model also facilitates cross-cultural care (Sohier, 1995). Permitting the client to clarify his/her comprehension of the problem, propose acceptable ways to take care of the problem, and accept a measure of responsibility for achieving goals places the responsibility in a shared context and allows a culture-centered view to emerge. This shared responsibility continues throughout the caregiver-client contact and is included in the exit interview and evaluation of outcomes. Specifically unique to the Neuman nursing process format is that both client and caregiver perceptions are determined for relevant goal setting (Neuman, 1995, p. 38).

Client strengths are often reflected in response to the question, "Have you had a similar problem before, and if so, how did you deal with it?" Evaluation of client strengths and weaknesses in the face of stressors assists the nurse in developing a client-centered plan of care. Occasionally the initial question, "What do you see as your greatest problem at this moment?" produces surprising responses. The reason for referral of the client or the obvious need observed by the caregiver may not form the focus of the client's need. This type of occurrence challenges the nurse to recognize the client's perspective in order to facilitate achievement of long-term goals (Neuman, 1995).

Because wellness provides a central focus in the Neuman model, nursing interventions are conceptualized as preventions and the actions of the nurse as reconstitutions. Neuman identifies three types of nursing intervention, labeling all as preventions: (1) primary prevention—when a threat to health exists but no stressor invasion reaction has occurred; (2) secondary prevention—when stressor invasion has occurred and action is taken to prevent the state of disequilibrium from progressing to the point at which basic structures become threatened; and (3) tertiary prevention—aimed at reconstituting a system seriously impacted by stressors to restore the system to equilibrium, optimal wellness, or its stable state (Neuman, 1995). Interventions at more than one level of prevention may take place concomitantly. For example, the nurse may offer assistance at the tertiary level in terms of reconstitution of a health state while applying primary or secondary teaching interventions in an attempt to prevent a recurrence of the response in the future. Because optimal client stability is the goal of nursing intervention in the Neuman model, it is to be expected that interventions will consist of more than one type of prevention. The prevention as intervention approach (three types) is illustrated in the cases described later in the chapter.

CRITICAL THINKING IN NURSING PRACTICE WITH NEUMAN'S MODEL

Nursing in the Neuman model facilitates and requires critical thinking on the part of the nurse. A thorough assessment following Neuman's guidelines is essential to support the development of a diagnostic statement, determine the appropriate interventions, and evaluate outcomes. In using the Neuman systems, the nurse is concerned with acquiring significant and comprehensive client data to determine the impact or the possible impact of environmental stressors on the defined client system. This process fully explains the client condition, providing the logic or rationale for subsequent nursing action. That is, it provides the basis for a broad, comprehensive, umbrella-like diagnostic statement concerning the entire client condition from which logically defensible goals are easily and accurately derived (Neuman, 1995, p. 38).

The nursing process based on Neuman's model is an interactive process between the client and the nurse that requires critical thought on the part of the nurse. Following Neuman's guidelines and assessment phase provides objective as well as client-centered information. The task of the nurse is to synthesize these elements, interpret them according to the model, develop a comprehensive diagnostic statement, develop goals in interaction with the client, provide care in terms of the three preventions, and evaluate the outcomes. Evaluation of progress and renegotiation of goals based on the client experience are important elements in the Neuman approach to the nursing process. Table 7-1 illustrates the interaction of the nurse with the client in the nursing process when guided by Neuman's model. Nursing based on Neuman's model requires critical analytic thought and interaction between the nurse and the client before relevant nursing action can take place.

TABLE 7-1 Critical Thinking and the Neuman Nursing Process	
Nurse	**Client**
1. Approach client, introduce self, make some small talk (weather, etc.)	Allow client opportunities to respond and relax.
2. As verbal and nonverbal contact proceeds, nurse asks: "What do you think is your greatest problem right now?"	Allow client to explain problem in own terms.
3. Question: "Have you ever had to deal with this problem in the past?"	Allow time for response.

TABLE 7-1 Critical Thinking and the Neuman Nursing Process—cont'd

Nurse	Client
4. If response is "yes," nurse asks, "How did you deal with it then?"	Allow time for response. Note strengths indicated by response.
5. Nurse then explains to client that he/she will carry out complete examination and history so that he/she can detect all problems that exist.	Assist client to prepare for examination.
6. Carry out complete assessment and history in the five variables: physiological, psychological, sociocultural, developmental, and spiritual.	Consider the client's needs (e.g., modesty, disability, culture). Maintain a caring attitude.
7. While client dresses, collate data and reach tentative comprehensive diagnosis. Share diagnosis with client and ask for feedback.	Ask client what he/she thinks would help alleviate problem. Client clarifies perspective on problem.
*8. Use nursing judgment about need for immediate action or new appointment with client at earliest possible time. Provide telephone number where you can be reached. Reassure client. Respond to any questions from client.	Client and nurse mutually agree on plan.
*9. Collate all data and determine nature of stressors facing client (intrapersonal, interpersonal, or extrapersonal).	
*10. Consider client strengths.	
*11. Develop problem list. Prioritize needs. Develop long-term and short-term goals.	Client clarifies priority needs and agrees to goals.
12. Meet with client and discuss findings. Propose plan of care. Listen to feedback and adjust plan of care if necessary. Contract with client about ways to achieve goals, identifying role that the nurse will play as well as expectations for client. Make any referrals or arrangements necessary for client to proceed with management plan. Reinforce identified strengths. Make future appointment.	Client provides feedback on plan. Client considers making contract with nurse to achieve mutual goals.
13. Meet with client, evaluate status, discuss progress, praise achievement or improvement, discuss reasons for failures, and renegotiate as necessary, listening carefully to client's position. Propose new plan as necessary. Make future appointment.	

*Steps 8, 9, 10, and 11 take place out of the client's presence.

ASE HISTORY OF DEBBIE

Debbie is a 29-year-old woman who was recently admitted to the oncology nursing unit for evaluation after sensing pelvic "fullness" and noticing a watery, foul-smelling vaginal discharge. A Papanicolaou smear revealed a class V cervical cancer. She was found to have a stage II squamous cell carcinoma of the cervix and underwent a radical hysterectomy with bilateral salpingooophorectomy.

Her past health history revealed that physical examinations has been infrequent. She also reported that she had not performed breast self-examination. She is 5 feet 4 inches tall and weighs 89 pounds. Her usual weight is about 110 pounds. She has smoked approximately two packs of cigarettes a day for the past 16 years. She is gravida 2, para 2. Her first pregnancy was at age 16, and her second was at age 18. Since that time she has taken oral contraceptives on a regular basis.

Debbie completed the eighth grade. She is married and lives with her husband and two children in her mother's home, which she describes as less than sanitary. Her husband is unemployed. She describes him as emotionally distant and abusive at times.

She has done well following surgery except for being unable to completely empty her urinary bladder. She is having continued postoperative pain and nausea. It will be necessary for her to perform intermittent self-catheterization at home. Her medications are (1) an antibiotic, (2) an analgesic as needed for pain, and (3) an antiemetic as needed for nausea. In addition, she will be receiving radiation therapy on an outpatient basis.

Debbie is extremely tearful. She expresses great concern over her future and the future of her two children. She believes that this illness is a punishment for her past life.

NURSING CARE OF DEBBIE WITH NEUMAN'S MODEL
Assessment Data

The case history is considered in the Neuman model according to the five client variables.

Physiological. These variables describe class V cervical cancer—stage II squamous cell carcinoma followed by radical hysterectomy/salpingoophorectomy, serious weight loss (21 pounds), urinary retention, need for catheterization, and radiation treatment about to commence.

Psychological. These variables paint a picture of a very frightened young woman expressing concerns about her future and that of her children, with little support from her husband.

Sociocultural. Debbie has minimal education and became pregnant at age 16. She is a guest in her mother's home where she lives with her unsupportive, "emotionally distant and abusive at times" husband and two children. She has smoked continually and excessively since age 13. The home is described as "unsanitary."

Developmental. The Neuman assessment would evaluate Debbie as a 29-year-old woman and mother of two children with a life-threatening illness. A Neuman assessment requires consideration of the adult developmental tasks appropriate to a 29-year-old woman, wife, and mother of a family. It is also important to ask whether her psychological development is such that she will be able to assess problems and tasks that face her in an accurate manner and tackle them when she feels better.

Spiritual. Debbie is tearful and fearful and "believes her illness is a punishment for her past life."

Organization Of Data

The next step in a Neuman nursing process is the organization of data in relation to the five variables assessed, identifying the nature of each stressor described by the client and/or observed by the nurse. Several areas in this case study would require additional data. For example, it would be useful to know more about Debbie's mother and the quality of their relationship and about Debbie's children and the quality of their shared lives. It would be useful to know whether Debbie is a spiritual person and if she is or has been affiliated with a church. It would be important to know whether a social work consultation took place before her discharge from the acute care setting to avoid duplication of work. It would also be valuable to know if Debbie's husband is looking for work and whether he is discouraged or even depressed. These factors are important in the assessment because the Neuman model is a systems model. Systems models always propose that whatever occurs at the system boundaries (e.g., between Debbie and her husband) can cause disequilibrium in the total family system. In order to clarify Debbie's problems and her needs, it is useful to plot the information in a chart like the one in Table 7-2.

   This organization of stressors reported in Debbie's case history permits the nurse to establish an initial understanding of Debbie's needs and to develop a tentative priority list. This list, however, must be discussed with Debbie in order to be certain that these are what Debbie considers to be *her* problems. Then a comprehensive diagnostic statement and mutual goals and plans can be decided on. It is also useful to create a prioritized list of the problems from the nurse's objective perspective and again from Debbie's subjective perspective. The client does not always agree with the nurse. A hypothetical example in this case might find the nurse placing Debbie's physiological needs at the top of the list. Debbie, on the other hand, might place psychological and sociocultural stressors regarding the future of her children before concern for self. These discrepancies must be respected, discussed, balanced, and fit into a care

TABLE 7-2	Debbie's Stressors		
Stressors	**Intrapersonal**	**Interpersonal**	**Extrapersonal**
Physiological	Cancer: radiation therapy planned Nausea Pain Catheter care—danger of infection Weight loss Smokes	Catheter care	
Psychological	Fear about future	Fear about future of children Lack of support from husband Mother (no data)	
Sociocultural	Basic education Fear of effects of smoking	Unsupportive, sometimes abusive husband Responsible for two children	Limited income Husband unable to obtain employment
Developmental	Has two children First pregnancy at 16 years of age	Mother of one teenager:13 Mother of one preteen:11	
Spiritual	Spiritual distress related to past life and present state		Concern over past behavior related to societal norms

plan that meets with the client's satisfaction. The nurse who fails to approach the situation in this way has less likelihood of achieving the goals essential to the client's obtaining optimal wellness. Neuman describes optimal wellness as the best possible state of health the client can attain at any one point in time.

Neuman's philosophical view is wholistic. The idea of a client composed of subsystems that together form a system greater than the sum of its parts forms the foundation for examining the five client variables and then restructuring the data to form a whole. "The various interrelationships of the parts and subparts must be appropriately identified and analyzed before relevant nursing action can be taken" (Neuman, 1995, p. 11).

Problem List

The stressors listed in Table 7-2, when considered by the nurse, lead to the development of a problem list like the one that follows. This list would be shared with Debbie to be sure that these are her problems as she sees them.

1. Pain, nausea, serious weight loss; understanding of catheter care; unsanitary conditions
2. Fear—lack of family support, concern about children
3. Spiritual distress—possible fear of eternal punishment

The nurse might approach Debbie in the following way in order to clarify the problems and her priorities.

Nurse: Debbie, I want to help you to be as comfortable as you can be now that you are home. What would you like me to help you with first? What do you see as your biggest problem?

Debbie: Well, my life just seems to be one big problem now; I am weak and tired and sometimes I hurt and feel nauseated. My mother has to work so she can't help me, and my husband seems more distant than ever since I got sick. And then I'm so scared about what will happen to my kids. I don't want them to be like me. I want them to stay in school and I don't want them to smoke because I know that cancer and smoking are related. And look at this place—it's such a mess! I just turn to the wall and cry. I don't know what to do! I think I'm to blame for all of this. I ran around a lot and got pregnant when I was 16.

Nurse: Debbie, have you ever felt this way before?

Debbie: Well, sometimes when my husband was abusive and so on, but that wasn't the same.

Nurse: What helped you then?

Debbie: Well, you know I went to work then so I could get away from it. And my kids and I used to have fun and I'd get them to help me clean up the place. But I've lost so much weight and been so sick, they stay away a lot at their friends' houses, and I don't want them to smoke!! (crying)

Nurse: What would help?

Debbie: I don't believe (sob) I know, but if the place were cleaned up and my kids stayed home some more, that might help.

Reflection On Data

When the nurse compares these two sets of data, it becomes clear that her priorities and Debbie's are different. Of course, it is important for the nurse to determine whether or not Debbie understands the medications, is taking them as ordered, and finds them to be effective. In addition, the nurse should evaluate the state of the catheter, whether Debbie has been taught and understands good sterile technique, and Debbie's personal state of cleanliness. However, these concerns are obviously not foremost for Debbie.

Debbie is frightened about her life and the future of her children, and she has a need from a developmental perspective as a mother to have the home cleaned up in the hope that she will be able to experience some close time with her children. It also seems as if she wants to do some teaching to help her children to understand the dangers of smoking and the importance of education.

Synthesis and Analysis of Data

Applying the Neuman model, the nurse considers all the data and the available resources and decides that she will propose cleaning services for Debbie if she agrees. Since Debbie said her children used to help her in the home, the nurse considers some way to involve the children with the housecleaner so they can help in some way with Debbie's care. She also plans to request Meals-on-Wheels for Debbie, who is often alone during the day when her husband leaves her alone without food. The nurse wonders whether he can be taught to accept more responsibility to help. She makes a note to meet with Debbie's husband.

Although it is not clear to the nurse what Debbie thinks caused her illness, it is clear that she is spiritually distressed. It is important to try to find out who might help Debbie with her spiritual distress. The nurse thinks of a female pastor at the hospital who is very empathetic, and with Debbie's permission she decides to ask this person to start visiting Debbie.

Having clarified the nature and strength of the stressors, the nurse asks how interventions can be structured so that they will reduce the actual stressors, improve the client's strengths, and prevent the same stressors from causing disequilibrium in the future.

The three preventions are used to develop interventions for this purpose. In Debbie's case, all three types of prevention are called for: secondary and tertiary preventions to restore her to optimal wellness, tertiary preventions to reconstruct the family, and primary preventions to teach Debbie about self-catheterization and to teach Debbie's children about smoking and cancer, their mother's needs, and how to take care of their own needs in the situation. In addition, primary preventions are necessary to teach the husband about his wife's illness and needs. Secondary preventions could assist in repairing the husband's self-esteem, and tertiary preventions may be necessary if he is diagnosed with depression. The whole family is affected by Debbie's illness and needs to be considered in the health plan. On each visit the nurse will reassess the situation, evaluate the health of the protective mechanisms, and intervene as necessary.

ASE HISTORY OF HOMELESS WOMEN

The client targeted in this Neuman approach to the nursing process (nursing assessment, diagnoses, and nursing intervention) is a group of 16 homeless women, clients of a 22-bed shelter in urban Boston. The shelter has religious affiliations and is supported by state, local, and private funding. The philosophical stance at this shelter is to assist women to move out of a homeless state by increasing self-esteem and building skills that will allow them to become self-supporting, thus increasing their likelihood of success when job and housing opportunities arise.

The 22 beds are full most of the time. Only three or four clients are long-term residents; the others are transitory, often returning after failed attempts to resolve their situations on their own. The assessment of this client required patience and time. The same women were not always present. The Neuman approach provides ways for the nurse to focus on aggregate clients such as a group or a system and facilitates the evaluation of a changing structure as easily as a stable one. This assessment reflects the perspectives of a changing group with certain common features that identify them as one system over time.

Individual Neuman physical assessment of the 16 women was carried out over a 3-month period. Because the identified client is the group of women, these physiological data were pooled at the end of the assessment phase to provide an accurate objective picture of the health of the group. This objective assessment was then related to the psychological, sociocultural, developmental, and spiritual assessment also carried out in group context.

NURSING CARE OF HOMELESS WOMEN WITH NEUMAN'S MODEL

This case illustrates a situation in which the Neuman model is applied to the nursing care of the aggregate client. A group of homeless women using an urban shelter forms the focus of the application.

Assessment Data

Physiological. The general physiological status of the group was, as expected, very poor. All individuals showed signs of malnutrition, poor hygiene, and skin conditions. Most of the women smoked, and many reported substance abuse. Tests provided evidence of infectious diseases including tuberculosis and HIV and AIDS. Some women had seriously elevated blood pressure, and several were diabetic.

Psychological. The psychological assessment provided information about lifetime patterns of abuse; early sexual abuse, including rape and incest; self-abuse; and self-mutilation. Generalized depression or episodic depression was reported together with a corresponding mistrust of society in general and the people with whom they had contact in particular.

Sociocultural. The group was predominately white, with their origins in low socioeconomic families. Some were Hispanic, and a few were African-American. Educational status was generally low, with a predominance of school dropouts, but a few were college graduates. It was evident from observing the group that they felt little trust for each other and had distrust of most authority figures. Some had made attempts to become established outside the shelter but had not succeeded, and they blamed their lack of success on the absence of support systems. Some spoke excitedly about ways they could succeed (e.g., job and training opportunities) and identified greater support networks as missing links. Others expressed helplessness in the face of societal stresses. Because they felt little trust for each other, community bonds were not developed. Despite their common experience, they were not a cohesive group.

Developmental. The youngest person was in her late 20s and the oldest in her 60s. Many had never learned to trust, and others were very manipulative in their attempts to manage the system. The general physiological development of the women appeared normal.

Spiritual. All of the group members exhibited high-intensity spiritual beliefs and evidence of religiosity or superstition. They said that certain good behaviors would be rewarded by a "greater force" that "looked out for them."

Neuman's Assessment Questions

When asked what they saw as their greatest problem (Neuman, 1990), the women agreed that their number-one problem was "having no permanent place to live." Many said it was "being without a job." A few spoke of the lack of "safe spaces" and "the gentrification of the city's North End," which had reduced the number of available low-income dwelling spaces. Several complained about their inability to stay clean, about "dirt," and about "binging" whenever food or drink was available.

Homelessness is a state of being that confronts nurses with what appear to be insurmountable problems. Applying Neuman's model helps the nurse obtain a clearer picture of the "mountain" to be tackled and guides the nurse to develop a clearer comprehension of where to begin to overcome the problems facing the client.

Organization of Data

Over time, while assisting at the shelter, the nurse realized that although the ultimate objective of the staff is to assist the women with making the transition from the shelter into permanent housing and with finding jobs and that this goal is what many of the women want, other problems interfere with this long-term goal. Many of these problems require nursing action. Organizing the data according to the Neuman model helps prioritize those problems according to the client's needs and identify shorter term goals to help them solve their problems.

Table 7-3 presents the stressors of these women according to their intrapersonal, interpersonal, and extrapersonal nature.

TABLE 7-3	Stressors of Aggregate Client of Homeless Women		
Stressors	**Intrapersonal**	**Interpersonal**	**Extrapersonal**
Physiological	Malnutrition High blood pressure HIV, TB, STDs, AIDS, diabetes Hygiene, skin problems	HIV, TB, AIDS, STDs Hygiene	Malnutrition TB
Psychological	Abuse (residual and actual) Fear Depression Lack of trust Low self-esteem	Abuse Depression Lack of trust Fear of people	Lack of trust Fear of society
Sociocultural	Lack of trust Lack of skills	Lack of support Inability to trust those who do try to help	Lack of support sytems Society's cruelty Lack of job training and opportunities to develop skills No money
Developmental	Lack of trust Absence of self-esteem Lack of responsibility	Lack of trust Absence of self-esteem	Lack of trust in homeless Absence of self-esteem Failure in society
Spiritual	Fear of life and society	Common belief in "something" Superstitious	Inability to profit from religion because of lack of trust of society

TB, Tuberculosis; *STD*, sexually transmitted disease.

The comprehensive diagnosis is disenfranchisement from society expressed in homelessness.

Problem List

1. Individual physical problems
2. Generalized low self-esteem and lack of trust
3. Depression, fear
4. Residual mental health problems related to history of abuse
5. Lack of education and job skills
6. Lack of job training opportunities

Reflection on Data

Long-term goals

1. To rehabilitate and house all those who can be rehabilitated
2. Find jobs for those who can work

3. Find resolution in a permanent sheltered situation for those who cannot work

The long-term goals for the group were identified by the nurse after synthesizing and analyzing the data. When these goals were presented to the women, they agreed that the long-term goals would meet their needs and were in the correct order of importance. As in all nursing process approaches, Neuman suggests breaking long-term goals into shorter term objectives that facilitate the achievement of the end goal.

Those who work with the urban homeless are acutely aware of the low measure of success generally experienced. Many of the problems are virtually intractable, and few respond to short-term intervention. Nevertheless, short-term goals provide a measure of hope for achieving success. Those short-term goals formulated for this group of urban homeless women were as follows.

Short-term goals
1. Improve physical health of each woman
2. Increase self-esteem in all clients
3. Reduce fear
4. Increase skills
5. Assist in job search
6. Provide long-term mental health counseling
7. Find training for clients

Working with this particular client group provides a clear example of the necessity of approaching the task from a wholistic perspective. For example, without a reasonable measure of physical well-being, interventions will not help the women to increase their self-esteem and reduce their fear of vulnerability. Likewise, unless they are reasonably well, there is little chance they will be able to learn new skills or take up the challenge of a job search. Unless long-term mental health counseling is available, the women short on self-confidence will have difficulty believing in success or that anyone will give them a new opportunity to learn and succeed. The disenfranchisement from society experienced by this group of women and the odds they face require simple, open approaches.

Sharing the initial assessment material with clients required an educative posture. First, they needed assistance to understand certain facts about the process of rehabilitation: (1) that it is slow, (2) that it demands work on some aspects of self and society to accomplish the long-term goals, (3) that the shelter staff and volunteers want to help in the process, and (4) that they also must participate in the process.

The women were asked if they agreed with the problem list and whether they could see that their first priority might require a short-term goal for their physical and psychological strengths to be increased.

A general consensus was reached and the discussion proceeded to short-term goals. The details for a contract were drawn up. In order to achieve these short-term goals with and for the client, the nurse must intervene, applying all three levels of prevention.

With the improvement of the physical health of each of the women, the core is stabilized using tertiary prevention. As physical health improves, secondary prevention is brought to bear on the psychological and sociocultural deficits, which improves the women's chances of getting off the street. Eventually, new types of skills and education for jobs and survival success in the real world are added (primary prevention), while constant tertiary and secondary interventions based on an ongoing reassessment are tailored according to individual need.

Recognition that the women are buffeted by intrapersonal, interpersonal, and extrapersonal stressors, which together present a picture of total vulnerability, leads to interventions that contribute to an occasional success story. Some of the women increase their trust levels sufficiently so that they believe in the good intentions of the people who assist them and in the shared experience of their peers.

Synthesis and Analysis of Data

When the short-term goals and interventions are clear, the client is asked how and in what way she would contract to work on self with assistance from the nurse. The plan of care is a "working with client" plan; therefore if the client has ideas of other ways to meet goals and these are reasonable, the plan is renegotiated until the client can commit self to a plan or part of it (see Table 7-4). Owning the plan helps the client achieve the short-term goals.

Each intervention is evaluated for effectiveness at each contact. If the elements of the plan are failing, they need to be discussed and renegotiated until a working plan is constructed.

The actual proof of the effectiveness of the plan and intervention depends on reaching the long-term goal—in this case, permanent housing and job placement for the client. Needless to say, rehabilitation of homeless women with such complex histories and problems requires long-term effort and commitment. Some of the women will succeed, some will succeed and relapse, some will need permanent shelter in mental health facilities, and some will choose to live permanently on the streets, returning to the shelter for respite from time to time. There is no question that the flexible and comprehensive nature of the Neuman model assists in visualizing, organizing, planning and delivering the complex care needs of the client. The assessment of the five client variables and organization of the data as intrapersonal, interpersonal, or extrapersonal stressors offer a clear picture of the challenges facing the homeless women at the shelter and provide the information to develop a plan of care to reconstitute their personal health and strengthen their protective mechanisms.

TABLE 7-4	Plan of Care for Homeless Urban Women Applying the Neuman Approach	
Nurse	**Women**
1. Make appointments for doctor's care for each person.	Support each other in keeping appointments.
2. Arrange for beautician for hair care and hand care.	Keep appointments. Support each other in doing so.
3. Conduct group therapy directed at increasing self-esteem.	Attend group. Acknowledge each other's successes.
4. Provide foot care (nurse and students).	Request foot care.
5. Obtain women's commitment to stay clean (away from drugs and alcohol) while in shelter.	Provide support for these efforts.
6. Provide education on communicable diseases.	Attend classes.
7. Investigate skills training and/or job training or schooling possibilities for client.	Accept opportunities as possible.
8. Assist in job finding and house search.	Believe in possibility of success.
9. Provide (with staff) opportunities for fun.	Participate.
10. Commit self as long-term care provider at the shelter.	Acknowledge commitment.
11. Lobby for needed programs and opportunities.	Participate if possible.

CRITICAL THINKING EXERCISES

1. Conduct a Neuman assessment on a friend using the five variables and determine the stressors. Use observational, clinical, and cognitive skills. Evaluate client experiential background and strengths.
2. Organize the data into a meaningful, wholistic picture and generate a stressor list, identifying the nature of each stressor.
3. Develop a primary diagnosis and a differential or alternative diagnosis, and discuss with your friend.
4. Take the nursing care plan from a patient you previously cared for. Sort the data from the plan according to the five client variables of Neuman's model; classify the stressors as intrapersonal, interpersonal, and extrapersonal; and develop a comprehensive diagnosis.
5. Using the case history of Debbie and the Neuman systems model, identify and classify the stressors for her children and her husband.
6. Think back to the last time you became ill. Develop an assessment of yourself at that time according to the five client variables. Sort the stressors as intrapersonal, interpersonal, and extrapersonal to explore how your stressors may have contributed to lowered resistance.

References

von Bertalanffy, L. (1968), *General system theory*. New York: Braziller.

Neuman, B. (1974). The Betty Neuman health-care systems model: A total person approach to patient problems. In J. P. Riehl & C. Roy (Eds.), *Conceptual models for nursing practice,* (pp. 99-114). Norwalk, CT: Appleton-Century-Crofts.

Neuman, B. (1980). The Betty Neuman health-care systems model: A total person approach to patient problems. In J. P. Riehl & C. Roy (Eds.), *Conceptual models for nursing practice* (2nd ed., pp. 119-134). Norwalk, CT: Appleton-Century-Crofts.

Neuman, B. (1982). *The Neuman systems model: Application to nursing education and practice*. Norwalk, CT: Appleton-Century-Crofts.

Neuman, B. (1989a). *The Neuman systems model*. Norwalk, CT: Appleton & Lange.

Neuman, B. (1989b). The Neuman nursing process format: Family. In J. Riehl-Sisca (Ed.), *Conceptual models for nursing practice* (3rd ed., pp. 49-62). Norwalk, CT: Appleton & Lange.

Neuman, B. (1990). Health on a continuum based on the Neuman systems model. *Nursing Science Quarterly 3*(3), 129-135.

Neuman, B. (1995). *The Neuman systems model* (3rd ed.). Norwalk, CT: Appleton & Lange.

Neuman, B., & Koertvelyessey, A. (1986). *The Neuman systems model and nursing research*. Paper presented at Nursing Theory Congress, Toronto, Ontario, Canada, Ryerson School of Nursing.

Neuman, B., & Young, R. J. (1972). A model for teaching a total person approach to viewing patient problems. *Nursing Research, 21*(3), 264-269.

Selye, H. (1950). The physiology and pathology of exposure to stress. *ACTA* 12-13.

Sohier, R. (1995). Nursing care for the people of a small planet. In Neuman, B. (Ed.), *The Neuman systems model* (pp. 101-117). Norwalk, CT: Appleton & Lange.

Orem's Self-Care Deficit Theory in Nursing Practice

Violeta A. Berbiglia

"Nurses work in life situations with others to bring about conditions that are beneficial to persons nursed. Nursing demands the exercise of both the speculative and practical intelligence of nurses. In nursing practice situations, nurses must have accurate information and be knowing about existent conditions and circumstances of patients and about emerging changes in them. This knowledge is the concrete base for nurses' development of creative practical insights about what can be done to bring about beneficial relationships or conditions that do not presently exist. Asking and answering the questions 'what is?' and 'what can be?' are nurses' points of departure in nursing practice situations." (Orem, 1995)

HISTORY AND BACKGROUND

The self-care deficit nursing theory (SCDNT) is one of the nursing theories most frequently used in practice. Orem's dedication to the concept of self-care resulted in a nursing theory appropriate for present and future healthcare scenes. The earliest development of the theory occurred in 1956 (Orem, 1985). Orem's purpose was to define (1) nursing's concern: "man's need for self-care action and the provision and management of it on a continuous basis in order to sustain life and health, recover from disease or injury, and cope with their effects" and (2) nursing's goal: "overcoming human limitations" (Orem, 1959, pp. 3-4).

The concept of self-care evolved into a theory as Orem and colleagues discussed and formulated the concept into a working description of nursing. Orem's model supports nursing through three central theories:

1. Nursing is required because of the inability to perform self-care as the result of limitations (theory of self-care deficit).
2. Maturing or mature adults deliberately learn and perform actions to direct their survival, quality of life, and well-being (theory of self-care).
3. The product of nursing is nursing system(s) by which nurses use the nursing process to help individuals meet their self-care requisites and build their self-care or dependent-care capabilities (theory of nursing systems).

The significance of the utilization of Orem's model in practice has been explicit since the publication of the first edition of *Nursing: Concepts of Practice* (Orem, 1971). Early use of the theory in practice began with the work of the Nursing Development Conference Group (NDCG) (1973). The group initiated their adventure into theory-based practice by integrating the developing concepts of the model into their clinical teaching of students. As the conceptualizations evolved, they were incorporated into nursing care.

The reality of nursing was further addressed by NDCG members who were in positions in which they could assert control on nursing systems (Allison, 1973; Backscheider, 1971). Members of the NDCG valued their work in practice settings for supporting their conceptualizations and revealing the importance of the broad conceptualizations to structure practice. The Center for Experimentation and Development in Nursing at Johns Hopkins Hospital was one of the early sites for the development of the theory through practice. Later, in 1976, Allison (1989) implemented SCDNT-based practice in the Mississippi Methodist Hospital and Rehabilitation Center.

Gradually, theory development in the practice arena began to filter into a variety of practice settings. Patient education was addressed by Goodwin's programmed instruction for self-care in postsurgical patients (1979). Graduate students at The University of Texas ventured out to implement the SCDNT in extended-care services and found that the self-care concept was growth producing for the nurses and the patients and showed the potential for cost-effectiveness (Anna, Christensen, Hohon, Ord, & Wells, 1978). Underwood (1980) brought the concept of self-care into the area of psychiatric nursing.

The literature of the 1980s reveals numerous efforts that further established the SCDNT in practice. This was a time when the theory was being explicated for use with specific nursing situations and in varying types of practice settings. The efforts that focused on nursing situations often centered on how patients managed illness through self-care (Dodd, 1982, 1983; Kubricht, 1984; Whelan, 1984). SCDNT-guided practice began to thrive in many settings: hospice—implementation of primary-care and self-care nursing (Walborn, 1980); public health departments—administration and delivery of care (Walker, 1986; Marz, 1989); rehabilitation center—evaluation of patient outcome (Allison, 1989); and a cooperative care unit—fostering of maximum self-care in acute-care patients (Weis, 1988).

SCDNT-guided practice continues to abound in a variety of settings and situations. Discharge protocols for self-care and dependent care (Taylor & Robinson Purdy, 1989) and for specific populations such as the elderly (Kennedy, 1990) have been designed. Steele and Sterling (1992) recommended helping method-specific interventions that are conducive to discharge readiness. Prescriptions for specialized practice—such as transplant nursing (Norris, 1991)—and for the provision of culturally sensitive care (Howard & Berbiglia, 1995) are appearing. The trend toward community-based practice has been supported by further explication of the SCDNT for use with multiperson units (community and family) (Taylor & McLaughlin, 1991), interdisciplinary care systems (Taylor & Renpenning, 1995), and community-based case management (Holzemer, 1992).

The International Orem Society for Scholarship and Nursing Science (IOS) (Isenberg, 1993) provides a forum for the exchange of SCDNT practice models. A sampling of the practice models presented at the IOS's Fourth International Conference reveals the structure that the SCDNT provides in innovative practices. In Germany, nurses are becoming proactive in their practices and anticipating that the theory will assist in the transformation of nursing practice (Berbiglia & Bekel, 1995). In Thailand, family participation in patient care of the elderly is stimulated by the self-care framework (Intarasombat, 1995). In the United States, a clinic for homeless men uses Orem's five methods of helping to guide nursing practice (Orem, 1991, p. 9; Martin, 1995). In some healthcare institutions, innovative computer programming has facilitated a blending of theory-based practice and information systems (Bliss-Holtz & Sayer, 1995; Riggs, 1995).

This review of the role the SCDNT plays in practice evidences its versatility. A product of the post–World War II period, the theory will continue into the next century as a guidepost for the profession. The timelessness of Orem's theory, its practical approach, and the utility of the theory in decision making are essential to practice.

OVERVIEW OF OREM'S SELF-CARE DEFICIT NURSING THEORY

Nursing practice oriented by the SCDNT represents a caring approach that uses experiential and specialized knowledge (science) to design and produce nursing care (art). The body of knowledge that guides the art and science incorporates empirical and antecedent knowledge (Orem, 1995). Empirical knowledge is rooted in experience and addresses specific events and related conditions that have relevance for health and well-being. It is empirical knowledge that supports observations, interpretations of the meaning of those observations, and correlations of the meaning with potential courses of action. Antecedent knowledge includes previously mastered knowledge and identified fields of knowledge, conditions, and situations.

Orem (1995) identified eight fields of knowledge essential for understanding nursing practice. Seven of those emanate from previously developed fields of knowledge found in the sciences and disciplines: sociology, profession/occupation, jurisprudence, history, ethics, economics, and administration. The eighth, nursing science, is knowledge about nursing practice created by nurses through scientific investigations that yield an understanding of the field of nursing and provide foundations for nursing practice. The practical science establishes essential content for courses focused on nursing practice. Personal knowledge of self and the other provides a screen through which input about the other is objectified. Insights gained facilitate a reality-orientation to self and the other and contribute to the "giving" characteristics of nursing: care, responsibility, and respect.

Practice knowledge is systematized, validated, and conducive to dynamic processes. Dynamic knowledge leads the user to acceptance and owning of the theory (Orem, 1988). Allison (1988) noted the dynamic quality of the theory and commented that the SCDNT always keeps the nurse in an action mode. Orem (1988) emphasized that today's nurses must be scholars within the developing theory. In doing so, nurses are committed to an awareness of the relationship between what they know and what they do. From this awareness comes a healthy sense of professionalism.

Awareness is heightened by access to and ascription to nursing knowledge. Orem (1995) referred to two categories of knowledge in practical science: speculatively practical knowledge and practically practical knowledge. She indicated that the theories and conceptual elements of the SCDNT are in the speculative category, whereas the practically practical knowledge is more particularized. It is knowledge that prepares one to practice. Practically practical knowledge, framed within the SCDNT, prepares one to practice by organizing knowledge necessary for practice in accordance with actions and outcome.

CRITICAL THINKING IN NURSING PRACTICE WITH OREM'S THEORY

SCDNT-based critical thinking emanates from four structured cognitive operations: diagnostic, prescriptive, regulatory, and control. Each operation fulfills a distinct phase in the use of the theory. Sequencing of the phases may vary throughout the process in order to reassess and continue to prescribe and regulate the nursing system for the best interest of self-care. The operations are intended to be collaborative and provide the self-care agent or dependent-care agent input into the decision making. Table 8-1 outlines the critical thinking requirements for SCDNT-based decision making.

Diagnostic Operations

The first phase, diagnostic operations, begins with establishing the nurse-client relationship and proceeds to contracting to work toward identifying and discussing current and potential therapeutic self-care demands. Basic conditioning factors are noted and considered in relationship to a thorough review of universal, developmental, and health deviation self-care requisites and related self-care actions. The projected value of requisites is estimated. An analysis of the assessment data results in a diagnosis concerning type of self-care demands. Self-care agency is addressed through an assessment of self-care practices and the effect of related limitations and abilities. Personal characteristics such as intellect, skill performance, and willingness are evaluated. From these data, inferences about the adequacy and potential of self-care agency are made, validated, and treated as diagnostic of self-care agency. Finally, self-care deficits are diagnosed by reflecting on the adequacy of agency to meet specific requisites. In instances in which self-care agency is inadequate, a self-care deficit is stated.

Prescriptive Operations

In the prescriptive phase, ideal therapeutic self-care requisites for each self-care requisite are determined by reviewing possible helping methods, considering related basic conditioning factors, and identifying the most appropriate helping methods. Actions required to meet the therapeutic self-care demands are discussed with the client and designed for maximum efficiency and compatibility. Priority is given to those therapeutic self-care demands that are the most essential to physiological processes. Client and nurse expectations are formalized and recognized as supportive of continued development of self-care agency.

Regulatory Operations

The prescriptions that evolve are used in the regulatory phase to design, plan, and produce the regulatory nursing system. Factors entering into decisions about design include basic conditioning factors, effective regulation of health and developmental state, timing, assignment of actions, and degree of cooperation. Further planning specifies conditions for the

TABLE 8-1	Critical Thinking with Orem

DIAGNOSTIC OPERATIONS

Establish therapeutic relationship	Enter into and maintain relationship
	Contract to collaborate in identifying and analyzing existing/potential therapeutic self-care demands
	Assess for basic conditioning factors
	Review existing/projected universal, developmental, and health deviation requisites
	Estimate value and expected changes in value of each requisite
	Consider interaction between basic conditioning factors and requisites
	Identify and describe self-care practices
	State specific limitations and abilities related to practices
	Make inferences about effect of limitations and abilities on engaging in self-care
	Validate inferences through continued observation
	Determine adequacy of knowledge, skills, and willingness to meet therapeutic self-care demands
	Estimate potential for development of self-care agency
Diagnose self-care deficits (existing or projected)	Make judgments about degree of ability to provide self-care
	Inform client of presence or absence of self-care deficit

PRESCRIPTIVE OPERATIONS

Calculate ideal therapeutic self-care demand	Review possible helping methods
	Consider validity and reliability of each method in relationship to basic conditioning factors
	Identify most appropriate methods
	Review identified methods with client/family
	Explain to client/family the sets and sequences of actions required for selected methods
Design therapeutic self-care demands	Consider time-specific relationships between requisites, economy of time and effort, and compatibility with personal and family life
	Plan for adjustment in design as requisites change or new requisites emerge
Prioritize therapeutic self-care demands	Prioritize in this order:
	First: Those essential for life processes
	Second: Those that prevent personal harm/injury or health deterioration
	Third: Those that maintain or promote health
	Fourth: Those that contribute to well-being
Prescribe client role and nurse role	Identify what client should do, should not do, and is willing to do
	Determine potential for continued development of self-care agency

TABLE 8-1 Critical Thinking with Orem—cont'd

REGULATORY OPERATIONS

Design regulatory nursing system for prescribed therapeutic self-care demands	Take into consideration the basic conditioning factors of age, developmental state, health state, and healthcare system
	Provide for effective regulation of health and developmental state by setting forth relationships among components of therapeutic self-care demands
	Specify timing, amount of nurse-client contact, and reasons for contact
	Identify actions of nurse, client, and others
	Take into consideration positive or negative cooperation
Plan for regulatory operations	Set forth the organization and timing of essential tasks/roles responsibilities
	Specify time, place, environmental conditions, equipment/supplies, and type and number of personnel necessary
Production of regulatory care	Perform and regulate self-care tasks or assist client in performing self-care tasks
	Coordinate self-care task performance
	Bring about accomplishment of self-care that is satisfying to client
	Guide, direct, and support client in exercise of self-care agency
	Stimulate client interest in self-care
	Support and guide client learning
	Support and guide client through experiences in meeting ongoing self-care requisites
	Monitor and assist client to monitor self in self-care measures

CONTROL OPERATIONS

Observe and appraise regulatory operations	Make judgments about quantity and quality of self-care, development of self-care agency, and nursing assistance
	Judge effect of measures on well-being of client
	Make or recommend adjustments in nursing care system
	Determine if:
	Regulatory operations are performed according to nursing system design
	Operations are in accord with client condition and environment for which they were prescribed
	Operations are still valid
	Regulation of client functioning has been achieved
	Developmental change is in progress and is adequate
	Client is adjusting to any decline in self-care ability

regulatory operations such as frequency, equipment/supplies, and personnel needed. Throughout the production of regulatory care, there is a strong emphasis on development of self-care agency by using helping methods that encourage learning, increase feelings of well-being, and stimulate interest in self-care.

Control Operations

Evaluation occurs in the control phase. The effectiveness of regulatory operations and client outcome is estimated. Regulatory operations are evaluated for correctness and appropriateness. Client outcome is appraised for regulation of functioning, developmental change, and adjustments to varying levels of self-care ability.

ASE HISTORY OF DEBBIE

Debbie is a 29-year-old woman who was recently admitted to the oncology nursing unit for evaluation after sensing pelvic "fullness" and noticing a watery, foul-smelling vaginal discharge. A Papanicolaou smear revealed class V cervical cancer. She was found to have a stage II squamous cell carcinoma of the cervix and underwent a radical hysterectomy with bilateral salpingooophorectomy.

Her past health history revealed that physical examinations had been infrequent. She also reported that she had not performed breast self-examination. She is 5 feet 4 inches tall and weighs 89 pounds. Her usual weight is about 110 pounds. She has smoked approximately two packs of cigarettes a day for the past 16 years. She is gravida 2, para 2. Her first pregnancy was at age 16, and her second was at age 18. Since that time she has taken oral contraceptives on a regular basis.

Debbie completed the eighth grade. She is married and lives with her husband and two children in her mother's home, which she describes as less than sanitary. Her husband is unemployed. She describes him as emotionally distant and abusive at times.

She has done well following surgery except for being unable to completely empty her urinary bladder. She is having continued postoperative pain and nausea. It will be necessary for her to perform intermittent self-catheterization at home. Her medications are (1) an antibiotic, (2) an analgesic as needed for pain, and (3) an antiemetic as needed for nausea. In addition, she will be receiving radiation therapy on an outpatient basis.

Debbie is extremely tearful. She expresses great concern over her future and the future of her two children. She believes that this illness is a punishment for her past life.

NURSING CARE OF DEBBIE WITH OREM'S THEORY
Goal for Theoretical Guidance

The goal for the application of the SCDNT to the care of Debbie is to prescribe the type of nursing system appropriate to meet Debbie's self-care requisites. The system designed should provide the optimum effect in the achievement of regulation of Debbie's self-care agency and meeting of her therapeutic self-care demands. A revised version of Laschinger's data collection and nursing system design tool (1990) is used for data analysis and critical thinking.

Diagnostic and Prescriptive Operations

Table 8-2 places the data from Debbie's case into the SCDNT framework. A review of Debbie's basic conditioning factors, shown in section A of Table 8-2, reveals a young woman caught up in what Levinson (1978) calls "the thirties transition," a time to claim full adult status in society. However, Debbie is lacking the characteristics necessary for the transition. The effects of early sociocultural factors (limited education, teenage pregnancies) are compounded by adult experiences: an insecure family system of limited resources bound to cope in an intergenerational pattern of living while dealing with the unacceptable environment of Debbie's mother's home. Debbie's past history and her present illness represent negative influences that impinge on her universal, developmental, and health deviation requisites. Essential universal self-care requisites (air, prevention of hazards, and prevention of harm), shown in section B of Table 8-2, have been threatened by a history of smoking, inadequate relationships, and psychological dependency. Her advanced stage of cancer and recent surgery have taken their toll, physiologically and psychologically. In section C of Table 8-2, it is clear that Debbie's failure to meet developmental self-care requisites places her at risk. The health deviation self-care requisites reflected in section D of Table 8-2 represent requisites influenced by Debbie's basic conditioning factors and developmental self-care requisites. Limited resources, developmental threats, and weak self-care agency surface in Debbie's own awareness/perception of her health deviation self-care requisites. She is expected to perform self-care and undergo extensive treatment although she lacks the knowledge, skills, and psychological security to do so.

The nurse encounters Debbie one day before discharge and is plagued by the weak self-care agency shown in Debbie's healthcare history: early sexual activity, a 32-pack/year smoking habit, and a relative deficit in managing developmental self-care requisites. The goal is to make a difference in Debbie's self-care agency. Using sections B, C, and D of Table 8-2, the nurse quickly identified the therapeutic self-care demands and stated these demands in the nursing system design (Table 8-3) for discharge. There are four priority diagnoses that are indicated with asterisks (Table 8-3) and are discussed here. First priority is given to the therapeutic self-care demands related to (1) elimination (provide care for eliminative process) and (2) adherence to medical regimen (ensure

Text continued on p. 142.

TABLE 8-2 Data Collection for Debbie

A. Basic Conditioning Factors

Age (yr)	Gender	Developmental State	Health State	Sociocultural Orientation	Healthcare System	Family System	Patterns of Living	Environment	Resources
29	Female	Early adulthood 30s transition	Acute phase of chronic illness	8th grade education Teenage pregnancies No work	Dx Surg Rx Plan	Married Children at home (2)	Lives at mother's home	Unclean	Extremely limited Husband out of work

B. Universal Self-Care Requisites

Air	Water	Food	Elimination
32 pack/year smoking history	No restrictions	No restrictions Weight: 89 lb Weight loss (19%) Nauseated Phenergan (25 mg per rectum prn nausea)	Urinary retention Intermittent self-catheterization

Activity/Rest	Solitude/Social Interaction	Prevention of Hazards	Promotion of Normalcy
Pain, nausea Percocet (1-2 tabs qd)	Tearful Expresses concerns	Husband abusive Keflex (500 mg po qid)	Dissatisfied with home environment Dependent on mother Radiation therapy

C. Developmental Self-Care Requisites

Maintenance of Developmental Environment	Prevention/Management of Conditions Threatening Normal Development
Teenage pregnancies (2) Oral contraceptives for 10 yr Dependent on mother Husband emotionally distant	No breast self-examinations Infrequent physical examinations No hormone replacement therapy Educational deprivation Poor health Oppressive living conditions

D. Health Deviation Self-Care Requisites

Seeking Medical Assistance When Health Status Altered	Awareness/Management of Disease Process
Seeks medical attention infrequently for overt symptoms	Aware of disease No evidence of ability to understand/manage effects

Adherence to Medical Regimen	Awareness of Potential Problems Associated with Regimen
Will perform intermittent self-catheterization Will receive radiation therapy	No awareness of need for hormone replacement therapy No awareness of radiation side effects

Modification of Self-Image to Incorporate Changes in Health Status	Adjustment of Lifestyle to Accommodate Changes in Health Status and Medical Regimen
Views illness as punishment for past life	Concerned for future of self and children

TABLE 8-3 Nursing System Design for Debbie: Supportive-Educative

| Therapeutic Self-Care Demand | Diagnostic Operations | | Prescriptive Operations |
	Adequacy of Self-Care Agency	Nursing Diagnosis	Methods of Helping
Air Maintain effective respiration	Inadequate	Potential for impaired respiratory status related to smoking	Guiding and directing
Water At present, no problem	Adequate	Potential for fluid imbalance related to nausea	Teaching
Food Maintain sufficient food intake	Inadequate	Actual nutritional deficit related to nausea and cachexia of cancer	Providing physical support
Elimination Provide care for eliminative process	Inadequate	Actual eliminative disturbance related to post-operative urinary retention*	Teaching
Activity/rest Maintain balance	Inadequate	Actual activity/rest imbalance related to pain and nausea	Providing physical and psychological support
Solitude/social interaction Maintain balance	Inadequate	Potential for social isolation related to emotional distress and husband's distancing	Providing and maintaining environment that supports personal development
Prevention of hazards Prevent spouse abuse	Inadequate	Potential for personal injury related to abusive husband*	Guiding and directing
Promotion of normalcy Improve living environment and lifestyle	Inadequate	Actual deficits in environment related to shared housing	Guiding and directing
Maintain developmental environment Support increased normalcy in environment	Inadequate	Actual delay in normal human development related to early parenthood, dependence on mother, and level of education	Guiding and directing Providing psychological support
Prevent/manage developmental threats Manage/decrease threats by receiving appropriate therapy	Inadequate	Actual developmental deficit related to lifestyle and surgical loss of reproductive organs	Providing physical and psychological support

Maintenance of health status Promote health	Inadequate	Potential for continued alterations in health status related to inadequate health-seeking behaviors, financial status, and knowledge deficits	Teaching Guiding and directing
Awareness/management of disease process Develop understanding of disease effects and management	Inadequate	Potential for urinary tract infection related to intermittent self-catheterizations	Teaching Guiding and directing
Adherence to medical regimen Ensure adherence	Inadequate	Potential for decreased adherence in self-catheterization and outpatient radiation therapy related to no apparent patient teaching*	Teaching
Awareness of potential problems Understand treatment plan	Inadequate	Actual deficit in awareness of advisability of hormone replacement and management of radiation side effects related to no discharge planning	Teaching
Modify self-image to incorporate changed health status Adjust to loss of reproductive ability and develop healthy view of etiology of illness	Inadequate	Actual threats to self-image related to disease, treatment, and guilt feelings*	Providing psychological support
Adjust lifestyle to accommodate health status changes and medical regimen Plan for future	Inadequate	Actual self-deficit in planning for future needs related to resources	Guiding and directing

*Priority diagnosis.

adherence) because elimination is essential for life processes. Prevention of spouse abuse takes second priority in that it will prevent harm/injury. Last priority goes to the therapeutic self-care demand for modifying self-image. Although self-image is important, low priority is assigned to self-image–related therapeutic self-care demands because they involve only contributing to well-being.

Regulatory and Control Operations

The nursing system design, supportive-educative, was intended to return control to Debbie and ultimately strengthen her self-care agency. The design was supportive-educative because the prescribed helping methods were designed to support (not compensate for) Debbie's self-care ability, primarily through teaching and guiding. The regulatory operations assisted Debbie to perform her self-care within a unified system of care. The support and guidance promoted her interest in self-care and brought her unexpected satisfaction with attainment of specific universal and health deviation self-care requisites. There was a possibility that a partly compensatory system would evolve if Debbie were unsuccessful in learning and performing intermittent self-catheterization and the nurse had to assume that action. However, control operations revealed effective regulations. For example, regulatory operations for intermittent self-catheterization provided for a self-catheterization every 8 hours until Debbie had less than 60 ml postvoid residual. A routine urinalysis revealed no evidence of urinary tract infection subsequent to the self-care actions.

ASE HISTORY OF MS. DAVILA

Ms. Davila, age 64, is under the care of a home health agency. Because of rheumatoid arthritis, she has been mostly homebound for 6 years. The home healthcare was begun at the time of her diagnosis with type II diabetes mellitus 3 years ago. She is pleased to report that she has never been hospitalized—even for the birth of her two children. Since age 50, she has had her share of health problems: osteoporosis, intense arthritic pain and impaired immobility, diabetes, anemia, and a weight problem. Recent laboratory reports showed triglyceride 250 mg/dl, LDH 290, and RBC 3.65. Her Accu-checks are usually somewhat elevated, but the diabetes continues to be managed by diet alone. She is 5 feet tall and weighs 180 lb. Weight has never been viewed as a liability in her Hispanic upbringing. Good times are always associated with eating.

Ms. Davila dropped out of school midway through high school to get married. Now as a widow, she provides a home in the country for her son. Her daughter and grandchildren live in the nearby city. Although her husband left a small retirement fund for her, she relies mostly on Social Security income and receives healthcare through Medicare.

Home care has met her needs well and has minimized expenses. Her largest bill each month is to the pharmacy for Darvocet N-100, calcium, and monthly vitamin B$_{12}$ injections. She looks forward to the home health aide's assistance twice a day and the weekly visit of the registered nurse. These visits are a source of social contact, which she rarely has anymore.

NURSING CARE OF MS. DAVILA WITH OREM'S THEORY

A complete data collection compiled from Ms. Davila's agency records and a home visit is shown in Table 8-4. Section A of Table 8-4 reveals that Ms. Davila has limited resources, has changed her lifestyle to accommodate chronic health problems, and receives home healthcare. In Section B of Table 8-4, there are concerns for the universal self-care requisites of food (abnormal laboratory findings and nonadherence to diet) and activity/rest (pain and impaired mobility). Ms. Davila has become somewhat developmentally dependent (section C of Table 8-4). She requires assistance in food preparation, hygiene, and toileting. The relationship of her universal and developmental self-care requisites to her health deviation self-care requisites emerges clearly in section D of Table 8-4. Ms. Davila is nonadherent to diet, has not modified her self-image to include dietary precautions, and seems to deny any diet-associated difficulties.

Diagnostic and Prescriptive Operations

Table 8-5 presents the nursing system design. All three priority diagnoses (denoted by asterisks) are classified as second priority because the therapeutic self-care demands are related to preventing health deterioration. In Ms. Davila's case, the SCDNT proposes a supportive-educative nursing system (with a partly compensatory component) that is designed to individualize her care. The individualization of the nursing system was accomplished through the overlay of basic conditioning factors and developmental self-care requisites (in sections A and C of Table 8-4) on the therapeutic self-care demands. The expected outcome is health status maintenance, health promotion, and prevention of further health deviations through strengthening self-care agency. The helping methods shown in Table 8-5 foster self-care. As noted earlier, the nursing system design would benefit from the addition of a partly compensatory component to supplement patient agency related to food intake. For example, supervised, restricted eating times, although they would seem developmentally appropriate, would produce increased adherence to the American Diabetic Association (ADA) diet. If Ms. Davila becomes extremely nonadherent to her diet, the nursing system design will change to partly or fully compensatory in an effort to promote physiological functioning and prevent health deterioration.

Text continued on p. 148.

TABLE 8-4   Data Collection for Ms. Davila

A. Basic Conditioning Factors

Age (yr)	Gender	Developmental State	Health State	Sociocultural Orientation	Healthcare System	Family System	Patterns of Living	Environment	Resources
64	Female	Ego integrity vs. despair	Disability due to health conditioning	10th grade education Hispanic	Home healthcare	Widow 1 son, 1 daughter, several grandchildren	Lives at home Son lives with her Leaves home only for physician appointments	Rural Items needed for ADLs in easy reach: shower chair and safety bars in bathroom, wheelchair ramp	Social Security income Medicare Son makes small contributions Refrigerator and pantry well supplied

B. Universal Self-Care Requisites

Air	Water	Food	Elimination
Breathes without difficulty Skin warm, dry Normal color for client	Fluid intake sufficient No edema Skin turgor normal for age	Triglyceride 250 mg/dl LDH 290 RBC 3.65 2000-calorie ADA diet Does not adhere to diet Weight: 180 lb Height: 60 inches Calcium (1500 mg po qd) Vitamin B_{12} (IM q Monday) Accu-check bid (usually between 90 and 120)	Voids without difficulty Last BM 4/20, normal

Activity/Rest	Solitude/Social Interaction	Prevention of Hazards	Promotion of Normalcy
Requires frequent rest periods due to pain with ambulation	Isolated—homebound and decreased mobility related to pain	Requires reminders	Has good relationship with son and daughter
Uses wheelchair at home	Communicates with daughter by phone frequently	Needs instructions on foot care	
Darvocet N-100 for joint pain (especially hands)	Home health aide present 2×/day	Prefers to walk barefooted	
Careless scheduling pain medication	Nurse visits once a week		
Pain not completely relieved			

C. Developmental Self-Care Requisites

Maintenance of Developmental Environment	Prevention/Management of Conditions Threatening Normal Development
Able to feed self once meals are prepared for her	Discusses condition and medical regimen with home health nurse and aide and family
Needs assistance bathing, grooming, toileting	

D. Health Deviation Self-Care Requisites

Seeking Medical Assistance When Health Status Altered	Awareness/Management of Disease Process
Reports to home health nurse any changes in conditions: blood glucose, pain, prescribed medications	Aware of disease processes
	Not compliant with diet or prevention of hazards

Adherence to Medical Regimen	Awareness of Potential Problems Associated with Regimen
Cooperates with medications	Aware of side effects of medications
Aware of medications and side effects	Appears to deny problems associated with nonadherence to diet
Aware of medical regimen	
Does not follow ADA diet well	

Modification of Self-Image to Incorporate Changes in Health Status	Adjustment of Lifestyle to Accommodate Changes in Health Status and Medical Regimen
Accepting of general health condition	Has adapted well to home healthcare services
Has adapted to limitations in mobility	
Has not been able to include healthy eating habits and weight loss in her self-image	

ADLs, Activities of daily living; *LDH,* lactate dehydrogenase; *RBC,* red blood count; *ADA,* American Diabetic Association.

TABLE 8-5 Nursing System Design for Ms. Davila: Supportive-Educative

Therapeutic Self-Care Demand	Diagnostic Operations		Prescriptive Operations
	Adequacy of Self-Care Agency	Nursing Diagnosis	Methods of Helping
Air	Adequate		
Water	Adequate		
Food	Inadequate		
Increase adherence to ADA diet		Potential for becoming insulin dependent related to failure to control diet and weight*	Teaching Guiding and directing Providing psychological support
Elimination	Adequate		
Activity/Rest	Inadequate		
Cope with/manage pain on ambulation		Ineffective pain control related to no real schedule for analgesic	Teaching Guiding and directing
Solitude/social interaction	Adequate	Potential for social isolation related to solitary living arrangements	Providing psychological support
Continue to maintain family, social, and home care contacts			
Prevention of hazards	Inadequate	Potential for diabetic foot problems related to carelessness in using shoes Potential for falls and fractures related to rheumatoid arthritis, osteoporosis, and obesity	Teaching Guiding and directing Providing physical support
Maintain safe ambulation			
Promotion of normalcy	Adequate		
Maintain developmental environment	Inadequate	Potential for deterioration of health status related to any future discontinuing of home health service*	Guiding and directing Providing psychological support
Continue to receive home health-care assistance			
Prevent/manage developmental threats	Adequate	Potential for misunderstandings related to mixed messages	Providing/maintaining environment that supports personal development
Keep communication lines open and clear with providers			

Maintenance of health status			
Awareness/management of disease process	Adequate Inadequate	Potential for diabetic complications, falls, and decreased mobility related to 3 chronic health problems*	Teaching Guiding and directing Providing physical support Providing/maintaining environment that supports personal development
Increase understanding of interrelationships of disease processes, diet, and hazards			
Adherence to medical regimen	Inadequate	Nonadherence to ADA diet related to lifestyle, motivation, and knowledge deficits	Teaching Guiding and directing Providing psychological support Acting for or doing for another
Increase adherence to ADA diet		Inadequate pain relief related to timing of analgesic	
Regulate administration of analgesic		Self-care deficit related to inability to inject medications	
Continue routine medications			
Awareness of potential problems	Inadequate	Potential for exacerbations and increased disability related to knowledge deficits concerning problems	Teaching Guiding and directing
Gain better understanding of cause/prevention of problems			
Modify self-image to incorporate changed health status	Inadequate	Inability to maintain ideal body weight related to lifestyle, motivation, and knowledge deficits	Providing psychological support Teaching Guiding and directing
Attain ideal body weight			
Adjust lifestyle to accommodate health status changes and medical regimen	Inadequate	Inability to maintain ideal body weight related to cultural attitudes toward eating and weight gain and meal preparation by aide	Providing/maintaining environment that supports personal development
Adjust eating habits			

ADA, American Diabetic Association.
*Priority diagnosis.

Regulatory and Control Operations

The SCDNT has been found to be especially useful in cases in which multiple chronic illnesses and medically prescribed interventions existed, such as the case of Ms. Davila. The theory guided the operations away from disease to the strengths/weaknesses of the self-care agent. In section C of Table 8-4, it is evident that Ms. Davila does seek to prevent/manage conditions threatening her development, yet she requires assistance in this area. The most significant self-care deficits are related to food. Section D of Table 8-4 shows that just under one half of the health deviation self-care requisites involved food in some way.

The theory also guided the nurse to analyze the self-care agency from the perspective of the basic conditioning factors. Culturally, we know it is common and socially acceptable for a Hispanic woman to be overweight, center her needs on caring for her family, and become more sedentary and gain weight at this age. So, although the nurse-developed supportive-educative system may appear to be a successful way to intervene, a closer look should be taken at the adequacy of the self-care agent and the potential for Ms. Davila to actually become motivated to alter her food-related habits. Are there motivators that will strengthen her agency? Is it possible to alter sociocultural views at this late time in her life?

The theory guidance provides an ample framework and fosters maintenance through the nursing system. However, it is evident that much of the responsibility for prevention and health promotion rests in Ms. Davila's hands. So, in retrospect, it becomes imperative to further analyze her developmental self-care requisites (section C of Table 8-4), prescribe and regulate helping methods that center on the maintenance of the appropriate developmental environment, and—at the same time—prescribe a system that is partly compensatory in the area of food requirements.

The extensive diagnostic operations in this case led to an important recognition. Do not expect one type of nursing system design to fit *all* therapeutic self-care demands. Plan at the beginning to supplement patient agency when faced with overbearing basic conditioning factors and/or problematic developmental self-care demands. This insight prevents wasted time, energy and expense; is more reality based; and places more responsibility on the nurse agency.

CRITICAL THINKING EXERCISES

1. The hospital where you are assistant nurse manager for the inpatient medical unit is revising the patient information booklet. Your responsibility is to develop a succinct statement of the nursing framework (SCDNT) that guides overall care at the hospital. Develop this statement using the outline provided by the vice-president for nursing. Remember, this statement is for *lay persons*.

   Outline
   I. Overall goal of nursing
   II. Five premises concerning the self-evident characteristics of human beings being served
   III. Three subtheories (self-care, self-care deficit, and nursing systems)
   IV. Nursing: helping methods
   V. Attainment of therapeutic self-care requisites

2. Nurses in your unit perceived you as a resource person on the use of the SCDNT and have included in the annual inservice program schedule an inservice program on the theory to be presented by you. The title they suggest is "Inherent Values in Utilizing Self-Care Deficit Nursing Theory in Inpatient Settings." As you develop the inservice program outline, what are the six values you list?

3. Looking back at the case study on Debbie, reconsider the basic conditioning factors. Which one do you think influenced her current health status the most? If that one factor could have been changed early in her life, what predictable changes in Debbie's self-care agency would have been possible? Project the ways that altered self-care agency would have prevented/limited the health deviations Debbie is experiencing now.

4. Mr. and Mrs. Cowan, parents of a 27-year-old man who is receiving inpatient rehabilitation for extensive burns incurred in an offshore oil rig fire, have an appointment scheduled with you to discuss their son's nursing care. Their major complaint is, "We are paying over $1000 a day for his rehabilitation! Why don't the nurses do more for him? He is so unfortunate and needs all the help he can get here." With the five-point outline presented above, you use your understanding of the SCDNT to reply.

5. James, an 8-year-old boy, faces a lengthy hospitalization as the result of recent injuries in a private plane crash. Both of his parents died in the crash. He has multiple fractures but luckily no neurological deficits. Identify three health deviation therapeutic self-care demands for James. Plan for these in a way that methods of helping will assist him to meet his developmental self-care requisites.

6. As you design the nursing system for James, do you perceive the nurse to be providing dependent care? If so, what factors in the nursing system indicate this?

Continued.

CRITICAL THINKING EXERCISES

7. Recently you were appointed to the cost-effectiveness department of a home health agency that is facing nursing fee reorganization. Explain to the department leaders the validity/reliability of designing a fee structure that utilizes a SCDNT framework. Explain how the fee structure can vary by nursing system design and specific helping methods.

8. Your high school class reunion will occur this summer. The reunion organizer has requested that each graduate develop a brief personal history to share with the class. Which of your basic conditioning factors are you most likely to keep a secret? What universal self-care requisites do you think they would find interesting? Which developmental self-care requisite do you especially want to explain to the class? Have a great class reunion!

The author wishes to thank Irma Lopez, B.S.N., R.N., who assisted with data collection and nursing system design for the case of Ms. Davila.

References

Allison, S. E. (1973). A framework for nursing action in a nurse-conducted diabetic management clinic. *Journal of Nursing Administration, 3*(4), 53-60.

Allison, S. E. (1988, June). *Making theory-based practice work: An administrator's view.* Paper presented at the meeting of the Self-Care Deficit Theory Institute, Vancouver, British Columbia.

Allison, S. E. (1989). Patient outcomes identified through theory-based practice. *Clinical and Cultural Dimensions Around the World* (pp. 147-156). Columbia, MO: Curators of the University of Missouri.

Anna, D. J., Christensen, D. G., Hohon, S. A., Ord, L., & Wells, S. R. (1978). Implementing Orem's conceptual framework. *Journal of Nursing Administration, 4*, 8-11.

Backscheider, J. E. (1971). The use of self as the essence of clinical supervision in ambulatory patient care. *Nursing Clinics of North America, 6*, 53-60.

Berbiglia, V. A., & Bekel, G. (1995, February). *The changing face of nursing in Germany: How can self-care deficit nursing theory assist in the transformation?* Paper presented at the meeting of the Fourth International Self-Care Deficit Nursing Theory Conference, San Antonio, TX.

Bliss-Holtz, J., & Sayer, P. (1995, February). *ISAAC: A theory-based information system.* Paper presented at the meeting of the Fourth International Self-Care Deficit Nursing Theory Conference, San Antonio, TX.

Dodd, M. J. (1982). Assessing patient self-care for side-effects of cancer chemotherapy—Part I. *Cancer Nursing, 5*, 447-451.

Dodd, M. J. (1983). Self-care for side-effects in cancer chemotherapy: An assessment of nursing interventions—Part II. *Cancer Nursing, 6*, 63-67.

Goodwin, J. O. (1979). Programmed instruction for self-care following pulmonary surgery. *International Journal of Nursing, 16*(1), 29-38.

Holzemer, W. L. (1992). Linking primary health care and self-care through case management. *International Nursing Review, 39*(3), 83-89.

Howard, J., & Berbiglia, V. A. (1995). *Caring for childbearing Korean women: A self-care perspective.* Manuscript submitted for publication.

Intarasombat, P. (1995, February). *Promoting family participation in healthcare for the hospitalized elderly.* Poster session presented at the meeting of the Fourth International Self-Care Deficit Nursing Theory Conference, San Antonio, TX.

Isenberg, M. (1993). From the president. *The International Orem Society Newsletter, I,* 1.

Kennedy, L. M. (1990). *The effectiveness of self-care medication education protocol on the home medication behaviors of recently hospitalized elderly.* Unpublished doctoral dissertation, The University of Texas, Austin.

Kubricht, D. W. (1984). Therapeutic self-care demands expressed by outpatients receiving external radiation therapy. *Cancer Nursing, 7,* 43-51.

Laschinger, H. S. (1990). Helping students apply a nursing conceptual framework in a clinical setting. *Nurse Educator, 5*(3), 20-24.

Levinson, D. J. (1978). *The seasons of a man's life.* New York: Alfred A. Knopf.

Martin, B. (1995, February). *Promoting self-care behaviors with clients who are homeless.* Paper presented at the meeting of the Fourth International Self-Care Deficit Nursing Theory Conference, San Antonio, TX.

Marz, C. E. (1989). New York referral intake and disposition: An application of Orem's classification of nursing situations. *Clinical and Cultural Dimensions Around the World* (pp. 107-126). Columbia, MO: Curators of the University of Missouri.

Norris, N. G. (1991). Applying Orem's theory to long-term care of adolescent transplant recipients. *Anna Journal, 18*(1), 45-47.

Nursing Development Conference Group. (1973). *Concept formalization in nursing: Process and product.* Boston: Little, Brown.

Orem, D. E. (1959). *Guides for developing curriculum for the education of practical nurses.* Washington, DC: US Government Printing Office.

Orem, D. E. (1971). *Nursing: concepts of practice* (1st ed.). New York: McGraw-Hill.

Orem, D. E. (1985). *Nursing: concepts of practice* (3rd ed.). New York: McGraw-Hill.

Orem, D. E. (1988, June). *Changes in the nursing profession associated with nurses' use of the self-care deficit nursing theory.* Paper presented at the meeting of the Self-Care Deficit Theory Institute, Vancouver, British Columbia, Canada.

Orem, D. E. (1991). *Nursing: concepts of practice* (4th ed.). St. Louis: Mosby.

Orem, D. E. (1995). *Nursing: concepts of practice* (5th ed.). St. Louis: Mosby.

Riggs, J. (1995, February). *Blending theory-based practice and computerization: The planning phase.* Poster session presented at the meeting of the Fourth International Self-Care Deficit Nursing Theory Conference, San Antonio, TX.

Steele, N. F., & Sterling, Y. M. (1992). Application of the case study design: Nursing interventions for discharge readiness. *Clinical Nurse Specialist, 6*(2), 79-84.

Taylor, S. G., & McLaughlin, K. E. (1991). Orem's general theory and community nursing. *Nursing Science Quarterly, 4,* 153-160.

Taylor, S. G., & Robinson Purdy, A. U. (1989). Assessing self-management and dependent care capabilities of hospitalized adults and caregivers in preparation for discharge. *Clinical and Cultural Dimensions Around the World* (pp. 4-16). Columbia, MO: Curators of the University of Missouri.

Taylor, S. G., & Renpenning, K. (1995). The practice of nursing in multiperson situations, family and community. In D. E. Orem (Ed.), *Nursing: Concepts of practice* (5th ed., pp. 348-380). St. Louis: Mosby.

Underwood, P. (1980). Facilitating self-care. In P. Pothier (Ed.), *Psychiatric nursing: A basic text* (pp. 115-144). Boston: Little, Brown.

Walborn, K. A. (1980). A nursing model for hospice: Primary and self-care nursing. *Nursing Clinics of North America, 15*(1), 205-217.

Walker, D. M. (1986). A nursing administration perspective on the use of Orem's self-care deficit nursing theory. In M. E. Parker (Ed.), *Patterns of nursing theories in practice* (pp. 252-263). New York: National League for Nursing.

Weis, A. (1988). Cooperative care: An application of Orem's self-care theory. *Patient Education and Counseling, 11,* 141-146.

Whelan, E. G. (1984). Analysis and application of Dorothea Orem's self-care practice model. *Journal of Nursing Education, 23*(8), 342-345.

Rogers' Science of Unitary Human Beings in Nursing Practice

Kaye Bultemeier

"Nursing is both a science and art. The uniqueness of nursing, like that of any other science, lies in the phenomenon central to its focus. Nurses' long-established concern with people and the world they live in is a natural forerunner of an organized abstract system encompassing people and their environments. The irreducible nature of individuals is different from the sum of the parts. The integralness of people and environment that coordinate with a multidimensional universe of open systems points to a new paradigm: the identity of nursing as a science. The purpose of nurses is to promote health and well-being for all persons wherever they are. The art of nursing is the creative use of the science of nursing for human betterment." (Rogers, 1990)

HISTORY AND BACKGROUND

The Rogerian model is an abstract system of ideas from which to approach the nursing care of the unitary human being. Martha Rogers first introduced this model in 1970 in *An Introduction to the Theoretical Basis of Nursing*. The central concern of the model is the nursing of unitary human beings. Within this model, human beings are conceptualized as dynamic, constantly evolving energy fields rather than homeostatic beings. Variation is expected and embraced within this homeodynamic perspective. Rogers' model, abstract in nature, becomes the basis for theory development that addresses the specific nature of nursing in caring for the unitary human being.

Nursing is considered an art and a science. The science of nursing is "a body of abstract knowledge emerging from scientific research and analysis." The emergent knowledge is translated into nursing practice (Rogers, 1970, p. 86). From the Rogerian framework, nursing is a science and the term *nursing* signifies a body of knowledge. Within Rogers' model, several assumptions regarding the nature of nursing are evident. First, nursing science is an organized body of abstract scientific knowledge that develops from research and analysis. This science of nursing helps to explain the human experience (Rogers, 1970). Second, Rogers contends that nursing is a learned profession and therefore must be based on solid scientific information. Third, because Rogers' model is a theoretical model, it is the predictive qualities of the model that provide the foundation for outlining practice. Theoretical structures are formulated, which subsequently guide practice and research. Fourth, formulated knowledge is to be used creatively for human betterment (Rogers, 1970). Nursing knowledge provides the tools for the emergent artistic application for nursing care of the unitary human being (Rogers, 1970). Nurses use this scientific knowledge to care for and improve the lived experience of the unitary human being. Nursing is the creative use of nursing knowledge in caring for the unitary human being.

Rogers' model contends that the human being and the environment are energy fields that are irreducible and equal to more than the sum of their parts. This wholistic perspective differentiates nursing from other sciences and identifies nursing's focus (Malinski, 1986a). Within the Rogerian model, the unitary human being and the environment are integral and therefore are viewed as a whole.

Nursing's focus is the care of people and the life process of human beings. Therefore its purpose is to identify and examine the phenomenon central to its concern, the unitary human being, and make predictions regarding human field evolution (Malinski, 1986c). Nursing aims to assist people in achieving their maximum health potential. Maintenance and promotion of health, prevention of disease, nursing diagnosis, intervention, and rehabilitation encompass the scope of nursing (Rogers, 1970). "Professional practice in nursing seeks to promote symphonic interaction between human and environmental fields, to strengthen the integrity of the human field, and to direct and redirect patterning of the human and environment fields for realization of maximum health potential" (Rogers, 1970, p. 122).

The life process of the unitary human being is one of wholeness, of continuity, of dynamic and creative change. Within the Rogerian model, the concepts of health and illness are viewed as pattern manifestations. Health for the unitary human being signifies an irreducible human field pattern manifestation (Rogers, 1986). The manifestation of health emerges from the mutual, simultaneous pattern process of the human and environmental fields. This manifestation is an expression of the process of life as defined by individuals and their cultures (Rogers, 1970). Therefore what we know as health and illness are continuous expressions of the life process. The goal of nursing is to help unitary human beings reach maximum potential. Clients define what is health for them and then nurses assist them in their movement toward that goal.

OVERVIEW OF ROGERS' SCIENCE OF UNITARY HUMAN BEINGS

Rogers' conceptual model is an abstraction that provides a way of viewing the unitary human being. Humans are viewed as integral with the universe. The unitary human being and the environment are one, not dichotomous. Nursing, within Rogers' model, focuses on people and the manifestations that emerge from the mutual human/environmental field process. Change in pattern and organization of the human field and the environmental field is propagated by waves. The manifestations of field patterning that emerge are observable events (Rogers, 1992). The identification of patterns that characterize a phenomenon provide knowledge and understanding of the human experience (Rogers, 1970). Basic characteristics are proposed and describe the life process in humans: energy field, openness, pattern, and pandimensionality. Other concepts that provide clarity to the basic precepts of the Rogerian model include unitary human being, environment, and homeodynamic principles.

Energy Field

The energy field is the conceptual boundary of all that is. The energy field is the fundamental unit of both the living and the nonliving. This energy field "provides a way to perceive people and their environment as irreducible wholes" (Rogers, 1986, p. 4). The energy field continuously varies in intensity, density, and extent.

Openness

The human field and the environmental field are constantly exchanging energy. There are no boundaries or barriers that inhibit energy flow between fields (Rogers, 1970).

Pattern

Pattern is defined as the distinguishing characteristic of an energy field perceived as a single wave. "Pattern is an abstraction and it gives identity to the field" (Rogers, 1986).

Pandimensionality

Pandimensionality is defined as "a nonlinear domain without spatial or temporal attributes" (Rogers, 1990, p. 7). The parameters that human beings use in language to describe events are arbitrary. The present is relative; there is no temporal ordering of lives.

Unitary Human Being

A unitary human being is "an irreducible, indivisible, pandimensional energy field identified by pattern and manifesting characteristics that are specific to the whole and which cannot be predicted from knowledge of the parts" and "a unified whole having its own distinctive characteristics which cannot be perceived by looking at, describing, or summarizing the parts" (Rogers, 1992, p. 27).

Environment

The environment is "an irreducible, pandimensional energy field identified by pattern and integral with the human field" (Rogers, 1992, p. 27). Figure 9-1 illustrates the coexistence of the fields, without limits and boundaries. The fields coexist and are integral. Manifestations emerge from this field and are perceived.

Homeodynamic Principles

Rogers' principles of homeodynamics provide a way of describing, explaining, and predicting a wide range of events that are perceivable

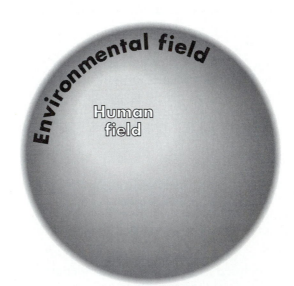

FIGURE 9-1

Conceptualization of human/environmental energy field. (From Bultemeier, K. (1993). *Photographic inquiry of the phenomenon premenstrual syndrome within the Rogerian-derived theory of perceived dissonance.* Unpublished doctoral dissertation, University of Tennessee, Knoxville.)

(Malinski, 1986c). Because the fundamental unit of the living system is an energy field, three principles of homeodynamics are proposed by Rogers: (1) resonancy, (2) helicy, and (3) integrality. These principles describe the nature of the person/environment process. The principle of resonancy embraces the continuous variability of the human energy field as it evolves. Rogers defines it as "an ordered arrangement of rhythms characterizing both the human field and the environmental field that undergoes continuous dynamic metamorphosis in the human-environment process" (Rogers, 1970, p. 101). Helicy describes the unpredictable, but continuous, nonlinear evolution of energy fields as evidenced by nonrepeating rhythmicities. The life process evolves in sequential stages along a curve that has the same general shape. Rhythmicities portend probabilistic predictions. "The principle of helicy postulates an ordering of the human's evolutionary emergence" (Rogers, 1970, p. 100). Integrality embraces the mutual, continuous relationship of the human energy field and the environmental energy field (Rogers, 1990). Change can be understood to occur by the continuous repatterning of human and environmental fields by resonating waves (Rogers, 1970). The fields are one and integrated yet unique. The principles of homeodynamics postulate a way of perceiving unitary human beings. The homeodynamic principles have evolved since introduced in Rogers' earlier works (Daily, Maupin, Satterly, Schnell & Wallace, 1989).

THEORIES FOR PRACTICE

The Rogerian model provides the abstract philosophical framework from which to view the unitary human being and the environmental field. Within the Rogerian framework, nursing is based on theoretical knowledge that guides nursing practice. Historically, nursing often equated practice with the practical and theory with the impractical. More appropriately, theory and practice are two related components in a unified nursing practice. Alligood (1994) articulates how theory and practice direct and guide each other as they expand and increase nursing knowledge. Emerging from Rogers' model are theories that explain human phenomena and direct nursing practice. The Rogerian model, with its implicit assumptions, provides broad principles that conceptually direct theory development (Figure 9-2). Theory can and does emerge from each of the principles, which directs practice. Two theories derived from Rogers' model are used in this chapter: Bultemeier's theory of perceived dissonance (1993) and Barrett's theory of power as knowing participation in change (1986).

Theory of Perceived Dissonance

The theory of perceived dissonance derived by Bultemeier (1993) from the Rogerian model provides a theoretical perspective for exploring situations

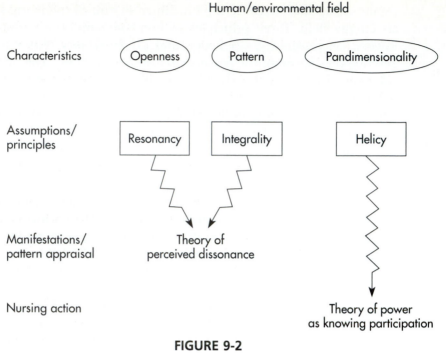

FIGURE 9-2
Two derived theories.

of varying resonancy as manifest in healthcare concerns currently labeled as abnormal processes. This theory emerges from the principles of resonancy and integrality. The theory provides a mechanism for pattern appraisal of manifestations of the human/environmental field during times labeled as "illness." The theory proposes that resonancy is altered periodically and rhythmically during the evolution of energy fields. The perception of dissonance during the rhythmical evolution of the human and environmental field is proposed. The theory of perceived dissonance delineates a human/environmental field process that is perceived as illness within the healthcare system. The theory embellishes and embraces the evolution of natural rhythmicities and manifestations associated with this evolution.

Persons are viewed as energy fields imbedded in their environmental energy fields. It is proposed that resonancy varies rhythmically during the evolution of natural rhythmicities. The inherent rhythmicity of fields can evolve into rhythms that vary and may manifest as discordant. During episodes of varying resonancy, the human and environmental field manifestations may be perceived as nonharmonic and as uncomfortable or unsettling to the person; thus the person views himself/herself as out of harmony or "ill." Likewise, others perceive the person as out of harmony or "ill." Personal feeling manifestations are identified that are associated with episodes of discordant resonancy.

Personal awareness of the emerging pattern manifestation is defined as being sentient to the evolutionary change of one's human energy field (Parker, 1989). A centered, receptive awareness is characteristic of integrality and is the means by which the person experiences varied resonancy, which may be perceived as dissonance or "illness." Alligood (1991) proposed that feeling attributes are a manifestation of the integrality of the human and environmental field pattern. Manifestations and feelings emerge, with discordant rhythms, that are associated with perceived dissonance.

The theory of perceived dissonance adds clarity to how the nurse can draw on perceptions by the client and have his/her own perceptions to provide nursing care. The pattern manifestations that emerge during times of variability, labeled as "illness," are crucial in providing a wholistic assessment of the unitary human being.

Theory of Power as Knowing Participation in Change

The theory proposed by Barrett (1986) of power as knowing participation in change emerges from the principle of helicy within the Rogerian model. This theory provides clear direction for the nurse providing care to the unitary human being. Within this theory, it is proposed that as knowledge increases, so does the capacity to participate knowingly. The theory proposes the capacity of human beings to repattern their human and environmental fields. This capacity can be used by the nurse and by the client during patterning.

Barrett (1986) describes power as being aware of what one is choosing to do, feeling free to do it, and doing it. "Power is a relative state characterized by the momentary continuously changing pattern; power is also a relative trait characterized by the more consistent organization of the human and environmental field pattern" (Barrett, 1986, p. 174). She specifies that the person must be knowledgeable for meaningful participation in the repatterning process to occur.

Within the Rogerian framework, the nature of nursing is based on theoretical knowledge that guides nursing practice (Rogers, 1970). The theories outlined, which are derived from the Rogerian model, provide the descriptive, explanatory, and predictive principles that conceptually direct nursing practice. These conceptual features have relevance to understanding manifestation for practice.

CRITICAL THINKING IN NURSING PRACTICE WITH ROGERS' MODEL

Critical thinking is a process of conceptualizing, applying, analyzing, synthesizing, or evaluating information gathered from, or generated by, observation, experience, reflection, reasoning, or communication as a guide to belief and action. Within Rogers' model, the critical thinking process can be divided into three components; pattern appraisal, mutual patterning, and evaluation. This chapter presents a synthesis of the two theories previously discussed and builds on the guidelines for clinical practice proposed by Malinski (1986c). In addition, Cowling's work (1990) assists in outlining the critical thinking process for nurses working within the Rogers' model.

Pattern Appraisal

The critical thinking process, as outlined in Table 9-1, begins with a comprehensive pattern appraisal. The life process possesses its own unity and it is inseparable from the environment. This wholistic appraisal requires the identification of patterns that reflect the whole. The pattern appraisal is a comprehensive assessment. Knowledge gained in the appraisal process is via cognitive input, sensory input, intuition, and language. The nurse gains a great deal of appraisal knowledge during the

TABLE 9-1   Critical Thinking in Rogers' Model

Nurse	Client
PATTERN APPRAISAL	**SELF-REFLECTION**
Comprehensive assessment of:	Nutrition
1. Human field patterns of communication, exchange, rhythms, dissonance	Work/leisure activities
	Exercise
2. Environmental field patterns of communication, rhythms, dissonance, harmony	Sleep/wake cycles
	Relationships
	Discomfort/pain
Intuitive reflection	Fears/hopes
Validate appraisal:	
1. With self	
2. With client	
MUTUAL PATTERNING OF HUMAN AND ENVIRONMENTAL FIELD	**PATTERNING ACTIVITIES**
	Meditation
Sharing knowledge	Imagery
Offering choices	Journaling
Empowering client	Modifying surroundings
Fostering patterning	
	PERSONAL APPRAISAL
EVALUATION	Areas of dissonance
Repeat pattern appraisal	Areas of harmony
Identify dissonance/harmony	Patterning activities
Validate appraisal with client	

interview with the client. Intuitive knowledge is gained from the patient as well as from the nurse. The client has self-knowledge to share. The nurse assists the client as he/she focuses on his/her personal patterns and rhythms. Using emerging pattern manifestations during the appraisal allows for a departure from the linear, cause/effect view. The nurse gains awareness of rhythmical fluctuations, with associated manifestations and perceptions. Patterning activities are based on probabilistic outcomes as they emerge from the appraisal of pattern evolution. The emergent human environmental rhythms and patterns are manifestations of the whole. Ongoing pattern appraisal, with multiple manifestations, can lead to prediction, patterning, and further pattern identification. The emergent rhythms are manifestations of the mutual process of human beings with their environments.

The client is encouraged to center and reflect on his/her personal pattern and the pattern of those with whom he/she shares common experiences. Pattern appraisal includes multiple lifestyle rhythms such as nutrition, work, exercise, pain, anger, depression, sleep/wake cycles, and safety. Another way to categorize rhythmicities is by utilizing the criteria developed by Kim and Moritz (1982). These rhythms include (1) exchanging (eating, elimination, breathing, giving, and receiving), (2) communication (verbal and nonverbal), and (3) relating (spacing, touching, eye contact, belonging, referencing). During the appraisal, special attention is given to rhythms of pain and discomfort or areas that the client is uncomfortable with or concerned about.

The nurse uses the feeling or sensing level of knowing, often described as intuitive or instinctual. The intuitive knowledge is best realized through reflection, which assists in pattern appraisal. The nurse realizes that manifestations are not static but partial perceptions of the synthesis of the past, present, and future. These perceptions provide the basis for the reflection and the intuitive knowing, which then further expands the appraisal. The manifestations, patterns, and rhythms are an indication of evolutionary emergence of the human field. Pattern appraisal and rhythm identification, along with reflection, provide the content for appraisal validation with the patient.

Mutual Patterning

Once the client/nurse have consensus with respect to the appraisal, then nursing action is centered around mutual patterning of the client human/environmental field. The goal of the nursing action is to bring and promote symphonic interaction between human and environment. This is done to "strengthen the coherence and integrity of the human field and to direct and redirect patterning of the human and environmental fields" (Rogers, 1970, p. 122). Patterning activities can be devised to address areas identified as dissonant and described as pain, discomfort, or anxiety. Through mutual patterning, manifestations of peace and enjoyment emerge (Lutjens, 1991).

Mutual patterning emerges from the appraisal and relates to areas of dissonance. Barrett (1990a) has outlined the components of the change process that are fundamental to formulating patterning processes. The components include awareness, choice, freedom, and involvement. Knowledge of the "disease" and various options for patterning are shared with the client. The knowledge shared is guided by the appraisal. Specific information relating to the "illness" and its treatments are included. The nurse must ensure that the patient has adequate knowledge of the appraisal and implications of various options. The sharing of the appraisal empowers the patient to participate in and direct the patterning process. Various therapeutic patterning activities are offered. Patterning activities instill hope and can be individualized. Modifications are made to allow the patterning activities to meet the limitations of the individual. The client must have the capacity to participate in the patterning.

The client is empowered by the process of patterning. Power is characterized by a continuously changing pattern. Power can be conceptualized as harmonious rhythmicity and a consistent integration of the human and environmental field pattern. The "goal of patterning is substantive change in health dynamic and change in the direction of health as defined by the client" (Cowling, 1990, p. 51). The nurse's goal is to assist the patient in reaching the maximum health potential and to assist in fostering harmonious patterns, thereby reducing the perception of dissonance.

Barrett (1986) defines repatterning as the continuous process whereby the nurse, with the client, patterns the environmental field to promote harmony related to the health event. "Change proceeds by the continuous repatterning of both man and environment by resonating waves" (Rogers, 1970, p. 102). Change is specific to an energy field and perceived through manifestations. Increasing diversity of field patterning characterizes the process of change (Rogers, 1970). Each human possesses changing rhythmicities that have individual uniqueness. The goal is substantive change in health dynamics and change in the direction of health as defined by the client. Without client participation, patterning is limited and evaluation is difficult.

Human field patterning. Patterning activities revolve primarily around noninvasive modalities. However, all treatments and interactions are patterning activities because they are integral to the human/environmental field process. Practice modalities concern human life patterning and reflect the wholeness of the unitary human being in "continuous innovative change with the universe" (Barrett, 1990b, p. 35). The health-related change modalities allow for change, they do not require it. Nurses currently assist clients in the use of meditation, imagery, visualization, and therapeutic touch where there is a primary focus of the patterning of the human field. Additional practice modalities based on motion, sound, light and color, humor, relaxation, nutrition, affirmation, art and nature, bibliotherapy, and journal keeping are also patterning modalities. The nurse is aware that the human/environmental field is one without boundaries. Awareness may center on the perception of the human field, but it too is a manifestation of the human/environmental field process. Centering is central to many of the modalities. With centering, the client focuses on his/her core or energy. This centering is perceivable as a harmonious field manifestation. The purpose of patterning is to "heal" the physical body or to modify the perception of dissonance. All manifestations, including those called illness, emerge from the mutual human field and environmental field process. The patterning activities help the client move beyond the physical body to pattern.

Environmental field patterning. Manifestations emerge from the human/environmental field process. The physical body is just one manifestation of the human energy field. The environment, with its healing quality, or lack of dissonance, is an important component of treatment. Wholeness implies concern with the totality of the human/environmental field manifestation. The key is interrelationship, energy patterns flowing through energy patterns. Wholistically, there is importance of the whole situation, background, or that which is relevant to a person or event. The nurse works with the client in the context of family, community, and cultural group. The nurse's concern for unitary human beings incorporates other nurses and healthcare providers as well as the nurse in the patterning. The nurse must recognize that attitudes, intentions, and feelings of those with whom the nurse works are an integral pattern in the environment. A supportive environment is needed for harmonious patterning. Color, light, sound, and smell are manifestations of the environmental field. These manifestations can be perceived as dissonant or harmonious.

The nurse, in consensus with the client, introduces a combination of modalities based on the pattern appraisal. The proposed patterning activities allow the client's health patterns to evolve or change to foster healing or a decrease in the perception of dissonance.

Evaluation

Evaluation is ongoing and encompasses a repeat of the appraisal process. Emphasis is placed on identifying perceptions of dissonance with respect to the initial pattern appraisal. The evaluation process is ongoing and fluid as the nurse reflects on his/her intuitive knowing. During the evaluation phase, the nurse repeats the pattern appraisal process to determine the level of dissonance perceived. The perceptions are then shared with the client and family/friends. Further mutual patterning is directed by the perceptions found during the evaluation process. This process continues as long as the nurse/client relationship continues.

Analysis and Synthesis

The Rogerian model provides a challenging and innovative means of planning and implementing patient care. The abstract ideas presented in the Rogerian model are fertile for fostering theoretical applications in the conceptualization of patient care. The unitary human being and the wholistic approach needed to provide care offer opportunities for nurses to design and implement healing environments that aid in the repatterning of the unitary field during times of perceived dissonance or illness.

Care for the unitary human being must begin with a thorough pattern appraisal that leads to a comprehensive analysis. The validation of this analysis by the patient is imperative before formulation of any nursing treatment strategies. Appraisal is ongoing and active. The client directs and assists in pattern appraisal. The nurse provides the synthesis and the conceptual understanding of the unitary human being process.

Patterning activities that the nurse introduces are instrumental in field pattern evolution. The patient experiences power as knowing participation in change. The nurse provides much of the knowledge that is necessary for this knowing participation, which becomes the springboard for innovative, noninvasive care of the unitary human being.

ASE HISTORY OF DEBBIE

Debbie is a 29-year-old woman who was recently admitted to the oncology nursing unit for evaluation after experiencing pelvic "fullness" and noticing a watery, foul-smelling vaginal discharge. A Papanicolaou smear revealed a class V cervical cancer. She was found to have a stage II squamous cell carcinoma of the cervix and underwent a radical hysterectomy with bilateral salpingooophorectomy.

Her past health history revealed that physical examinations had been infrequent. She also reported that she had not performed breast self-examination. She is 5 feet 4 inches tall and weighs 89 pounds. Her usual weight is about 110 pounds. She has smoked approximately two packs of cigarettes a day for the past 16 years. She is gravida 2, para 2. Her first pregnancy was at age 16, and her second was at age 18. Since that time she has taken oral contraceptives on a regular basis.

Debbie completed the eighth grade. She is married and lives with her husband and two children in her mother's home, which she describes as less than sanitary. Her husband is unemployed. She describes him as emotionally distant and abusive at times.

She has done well following surgery except for being unable to completely empty her urinary bladder. She is having continued postoperative pain and nausea. It will be necessary for her to perform intermittent self-catherization at home. Her home medications are (1) an antibiotic, (2) an analgesic as needed for pain, and (3) an antiemetic as needed for nausea. In addition, she will be receiving radiation therapy on an outpatient basis.

Debbie is extremely tearful. She expresses great concern over her future and the future of her two children. She believes that this illness is a punishment for her past life.

NURSING CARE OF DEBBIE WITH ROGERS' MODEL

Within the Rogerian model, the process of caring for Debbie begins with pattern appraisal. Pattern appraisal is the most important component of the nursing process. Nursing care will involve pattern appraisal, mutual patterning, and evaluation.

Pattern Appraisal

The history provides a beginning and a major portion of the pattern appraisal. Debbie has a pattern of smoking, which has been associated with less than optimal health potential. This visible rhythmical pattern is a manifestation of evolution toward dissonance. In addition, Debbie has a pattern manifestation that has been labeled "cervical cancer." This emergent pattern manifests as dissonant. Debbie has a low educational level, which is relevant as patterning activities are introduced. A pattern manifestation of healing is noted through reports of a positive operative course.

Sensory data add to the pattern appraisal. Through language, Debbie identifies a perception of dissonance with her husband and with her environment, which she describes as "unsanitary." The nurse will explore with Debbie what perceptions and feelings she has with respect to her home environment. Can patterning be directed toward a reduction in perceived dissonance with her environmental field? Pain is a manifestation that needs to be further evaluated to determine the pattern of pain perception. Appraisal of pain as it relates to circadian rhythms and environmental field changes assist in this appraisal. Debbie is asked to reflect on characteristics of the pain, and together with the nurse a pattern may emerge. Pain is a manifestation of dissonance.

The nurse has reported that Debbie has a manifestation of fear. Debbie reports the fear of dealing with her life after this illness, and the nurse senses this manifestation of fear. Debbie's self-knowledge links the illness to her personal belief of "being punished" for past mistakes. History and focusing on the "relative present" to explore the pattern of punishment is imperative. It is important that the nurse appraise the environment of the hospital and of the others who share her existence. Fear is a manifestation of dissonance and is reported by Debbie. The pain and fear are dissonant manifestations. Appraisal of human/environmental factors as these perceptions emerge is needed.

Language provides a valuable addition to the pattern appraisal of Debbie. Appraisal is needed concerning Debbie's sleep patterns, her nutritional status, and her perceptions of self and what is a healthful or harmonious existence for her. This appraisal can be grouped into exchanging patterns, communication patterns, and relating patterns, as discussed previously. Time between the nurse and patient is needed to foster this comprehensive appraisal of Debbie. During this entire process, the nurse must rely heavily on personal intuition and insight regarding the pattern that is emergent with Debbie. All of the knowledge gained forms the unitary pattern of Debbie.

Dissonance can be perceived in many aspects of Debbie's appraisal. There is a lack of environmental harmony as noted in the patient's perception of it being unsanitary. In addition, dissonance is perceived with respect to her relationship with her husband. Personal dissonance is noted in the manifestations of cancer, weight loss, pain, nausea, and tobacco use. This dissonance is also conceptualized as fear in the words of the patient and in the emotional distance that she feels.

On completion of the pattern appraisal, the analysis is presented to the patient. Emphasis can be placed on areas in which dissonance and harmony are noted in the personal and environmental field manifestations. Consensus needs to be reached with Debbie before patterning activities can be suggested and implemented.

Mutual Patterning

Patterning can be approached from many directions. The process is mutual between nurse and patient. The surgery is a patterning activity. Manifestations will evolve from the surgical intervention that will require reconceptualization and validation with the client. Medications are patterning modalities. Debbie is receiving medications. Decisions are made in conjunction with Debbie regarding the use of the medications and the patterning that emerges with the introduction of these modalities. Personal knowledge regarding the surgery and the medications empower Debbie to be a vital agent in the selection of modalities. Debbie possesses freedom and involvement in the selection of modalities. Options to entertain include therapeutic touch, humor, meditation, visualization, and imagery. Debbie needs to be assessed fully regarding her ability to understand and agree with different patterning modalities.

Therapeutic touch can be introduced to Debbie. The touch is introduced and incorporated into the management of pain manifestations. Touch in combination with medications provide patterning that Debbie can direct. The nurse can introduce the process of touch to Debbie's husband and teach him how to incorporate touch into her care. Another option would be to teach Debbie how to center her energy and channel her energy to the area that is experiencing pain.

Patterning directed at the manifestation of fear is needed. Options including imagery, music, light, and meditation can be discussed. Fear manifests as apprehension of self-catheterization. Emphasis needs to be placed on having Debbie direct how, where, when, and with whom the self-catheterization will be taught. Establishing a rhythm to the catheterization schedule that is harmonious with Debbie's life would reduce dissonance. Patterning of nutrition and catheterization based on the pattern appraisal can assist in empowering Debbie to learn self-catheterization. A rhythm will evolve that is harmonious with Debbie and her energy field rhythm. Specific actions of the nurse with respect to language and knowledge about the catheterization process empower Debbie to direct this phase of her treatment.

Human/environment patterning needs to involve the other individuals who share Debbie's environment, including her husband, children, and mother. Options are introduced relating to increased communication and sanitation patterns. The entire family is involved in power as knowing participation in change. Language and the use of language is explored to determine what Debbie would prefer to change in her environment and sanitation. Options are introduced that allow pattern evolution integral with her environment that is not perceived as dissonant.

Evaluation

The evaluation process centers on the perceptions of dissonance that exist after the mutual patterning activities. The appraisal process is repeated. Specific emphasis is placed on emergent patterns of dissonance that are still evident. Manifestations of pain, fear, and tension with family members are appraised. The nurse intuitively evaluates the amount of dissonance that is manifesting with respect to Debbie as he/she cares for her. A summary of the dissonance and/or harmony that is perceived is then shared with Debbie, and mutual patterning is modified or instituted as indicated based on the evaluation.

Mary is a 42-year-old woman who has been admitted to the oncology unit for pain management and testing. She becomes teary during the history taking and reports that she has had a recent recurrence of metastatic breast cancer and is here to determine future options for her care.

Mary is accompanied by her husband and two children, ages 15 and 10. Her husband and children appear anxious but supportive and attentive. She states she is employed as an interior decorator and is well respected in the community.

Mary reports that breast cancer was first diagnosed in 1993. Initial therapy included 6 months of chemotherapy followed by a mastectomy and radiation therapy. At the time of mastectomy, she was found to have axillary lymph node involvement of the carcinoma. In 1994, she underwent reconstructive surgery of the breast. At a routine follow-up examination 6 months ago, she was found to have two metastatic lesions of the spine and one of the hip and fluid noted around the liver. Chemotherapy was reinstituted. At the follow-up examination for the chemotherapy last week, she was informed that four new metastatic lesions had developed while she was on the chemotherapy and that her options are limited.

Mary reports that she has always remained hopeful during her journey with the cancer. She feels that she has learned a great deal about herself during her illness and has grown closer to her family and friends. After her initial treatment, Mary was instrumental in the formation of a local breast cancer support group and is currently the chairperson. She reports sadly that she has not been back to the group since the recurrence of the cancer since she does not want to discourage other members.

Mary has read extensively on self-healing. She practices yoga and does weaving as a hobby. Her response after the mastectomy was to invite five dear friends to share a ritual that involved burying her diseased breast (a plaster replica). She viewed this ceremony as a new beginning for her life as she prepared for reconstructive surgery. She denies any real spiritual orientation.

Mary has a trusting, comfortable relationship with her oncologist and sadly reports that recently she has entertained the notion of consulting someone new since the disease has progressed. She says that for the first time she is really frightened and willing to do almost anything that might give her more time with her family.

Mary's weight is 140 pounds and her height is 5 feet 6 inches. She takes medications for pain and depression. Her general appearance is that of a teary-eyed woman in no acute distress. She sits quietly on the bed holding her husband's hand during the interview. She is articulate.

NURSING CARE OF MARY WITH ROGERS' MODEL

Nursing care for Mary offers the opportunity to incorporate many variations in patterning activities. These patterning activities will be directed by the knowledge gained during the appraisal phase. As Mary nears and prepares for the end of her life, many patterning concerns must be addressed for peaceful closure to her life and the change to another energy form. The steps involve pattern appraisal, mutual patterning modalities, and evaluation of the dissonance perceived before, during, and after patterning activities.

Pattern Appraisal

The pattern appraisal has begun. Mary is verbal and intuitive. She readily shares with others the story of her journey with cancer. A sense of sadness and communion with others is perceived. Dissonance is noted in the progression of the disease, in her pain, and in her "confusion" regarding how to proceed and whether to remain with her oncologist. Harmony is noted in her relationship with her husband and family and with her sense of how she has progressed through this "disease" process.

Mary has a great deal of knowledge about herself and about the disease. Mary, her family, and the nurse are aware that the pattern of breast cancer with multiple metastases is one of eventual death. The dissonance of the cancer is a rhythmical emergence that is pervasive to her wholeness.

Sensory data are gained through language, feelings, and perceptions. The nurse perceives that much attention to sensory information is needed because Mary has a great deal to share about her feelings regarding the disease and her thoughts and fears. Dissonance is perceived through her acknowledgment of fear and apprehension regarding her future.

Intuition is a major source of self-knowledge for Mary. She relates that it is hard for her to accept that she is that sick because she looks so good and feels fairly good. She states that intuitively her body tells her that she will be okay. However, all healthcare providers give her an entirely different perception of her health. The intuitive knowing of the nurse is crucial in completing the pattern appraisal. Cognitive knowing tells the nurse that Mary's condition is grave; however, the addition of intuitive knowledge on the nurse's part may change the unitary perspective.

Knowledge gained through language is integral to the assessment. Mary and her family have a great deal of self-knowledge to share. Perceptions and beliefs regarding health and illness are important to the appraisal. Conversation with Mary flows easily and reveals a great deal. Mary is articulate and shares freely her perceptions of what is occurring to her and her family.

Valuable information regarding areas of dissonance can be gained through a field evaluation using therapeutic touch. During the initial examination, the nurse uses therapeutic touch to identify any irregularities of the energy field and also to channel energy for pain control. Energy field appraisal with assessment of areas of pattern distortion adds critical information.

The unitary image that emerges is one of dissonance that manifests as "metastatic breast cancer." The Rogerian model guides us to a field evaluation and analysis. Mary, her husband, and children are a field pattern. The objective signs and symptoms are merely perceivable field pattern manifestations. The diagnosis of metastatic breast cancer is the label that has been applied to the pattern manifestation.

Mutual Patterning

A sharing of the unitary pattern appraisal with Mary is imperative. Mary will confirm or reject the appraisal, and this appraisal will become the basis for the patterning recommendations. The nurse helps create an environment in which healing conditions are optimal and invites Mary to heal herself as she participates in various modalities used in deliberative mutual patterning.

Change is continuous and in the direction of increasing diversity of patterning. The varying forms of manifestation that are associated with change become somewhat predictable. For practice, this means a consideration of the manifestations relative to the individual in developing practice aims. As Mary deals with her emergent pattern, pain is a frequent perceivable manifestation. Assistance in options for the management of pain is needed.

The use of different-color light waves can be proposed to Mary. McDonald (1986) examined the relationship between visible light waves and the experience of pain. She reported that blue light waves decrease pain in rheumatoid arthritis sufferers. Trials of various colors and their patterning ability on the manifestation of pain could be offered. Mary, who is an interior decorator, has strong preferences/dislikes for various colors. Since the hospital walls are white, color can be introduced through blankets and/or sheets brought by the family. Mary can be asked whether she wishes to have certain art objects or flowers brought to her room. Every effort should be made to make the room environment consistent with Mary's preferences. Attention should also be given to the amount and type of light in Mary's room. Does she prefer natural, incandescent, or fluorescent light? The family can be encouraged to bring a bedside incandescent light if she prefers. The use of sound in the environment is also helpful for patterning. Mary is encouraged to have her family bring a tape player or CD player and music that she enjoys.

Therapeutic touch is introduced for assistance in the dissonant emergence of pain. Options are proposed relating to intermittent therapeutic touch. Modalities are taught to family members so that they can continue the patterning in the absence of the nurse or after hospitalization. The family needs to be assessed as to their comfort level with respect to administering therapeutic touch. Families can be easily taught how to smooth the energy field and how to direct energy to areas of concern/pain. Therapeutic touch can be helpful to Mary and to her family as it allows closeness and the ability to nurture Mary through her pain.

Living/dying is a rhythmic manifestation of the life process. Unitary human and environmental rhythms find expression in the rhythmicities of the living/dying process. Death is a very real possibility for Mary. The nurses caring for Mary are concerned with dying as well as with living. Dying is a developmental process, during which there is continued actualization of potentials (Phillips, 1990, p. 19). According to Rogers (1992), dying is moving beyond the pattern visible to human perception. Death is a transformation of energy (Rogers, 1970). At death, the human field ceases to exist, and identity as a living human being is gone. The process of dying is a period of transition in which the integrity of the human field as such diminishes and dies (Rogers, 1970). A transformation of energy occurs. As the pattern of cancer evolves for Mary, manifestations of pain will increase and the reality of impending death will emerge. Nursing care will revolve around the introduction of several modalities that may assist Mary and her family as the human/environmental field evolves.

Uninterrupted time for Mary and her family to be together is imperative. Attention to visitation based on the rhythm of Mary is implemented. Children, friends, and family can visit without restriction and are encouraged to bring items that help them feel harmonious in the hospital environment.

The power of humor in the patterning of chronic illness manifestation is proposed. Options include movies, books, or recordings. Sources for materials are shared with Mary and her family. Hospital volunteers are asked to search for and bring materials to Mary. Mary and her family are offered the option of bringing their VCR so that they may view humorous films if they so desire. The hospital medical library is consulted to see whether they have materials that could be used by Mary and her family. Nursing staff are encouraged to maintain their humor in their care for Mary. Often nursing staff members avoid terminally ill patients, and care should be taken to keep staff who are comfortable with terminally ill patients assigned to Mary. Mary is offered some input into who is her nurse.

Meditation is introduced as a form of centering for Mary. Mary is asked to focus on a quiet spot or a part of her body and slow down her breathing. She may choose to have her eyes open or closed. She may elect to center on a pleasant object in her room. Meditative music is introduced into the environment. Care is taken to place a sign on Mary's door indicating "do not disturb" during meditation time.

Medication is also incorporated into the care of Mary's pain. Mary has identified that she is much more comfortable if she takes her pain medication every 4 hours and does not wait for it to "get bad." A routine is developed to allow Mary to receive her medication every 4 hours routinely, and the family is involved in the administration of the dosage.

Mary and her family are close. The suggestion of journaling as a means of patterning her evolution into death is introduced. This journaling is used by Mary and by her family to record the relative present. This journal provides a forum for discussion of many issues regarding Mary's illness and her sadness regarding not seeing her children grow up. Nurses freely discuss their perceptions and share the joy they have in caring for Mary.

Mary is a professional interior decorator. The importance of color, light, and pattern are integral to her care. Options regarding how her physical space is oriented, decorated, and located are explored in the patterning of Mary. She and her family are given latitude in bringing personal effects, artwork, children's drawings, and photographs. The bed is turned to face the window at Mary's request. A favorite rocker and a bright rug for the floor are brought from home. Mary elects to place a beautiful cloth over her bedside table and has her small weaving loom placed in the room. The room radiates a sense of peace and the feeling of "hospital" is lost.

Evaluation

Recurrent evaluation and pattern appraisal is needed with Mary as she approaches death. Intuition and family reflections assist the nurse in their knowing. A complete pattern appraisal is repeated with special attention to dissonance perceived in respect to pain. Therapeutic touch is administered to identify any field irregularities. A temporal recording of perceptions that surround the "pain" is reviewed. Perceptions of dissonance are identified, verified with Mary, and new patterning modalities introduced. The care of Mary is most rewarding within a Rogerian model. She exemplifies a unitary human spirit that has been attuned to energy and intuition her entire life.

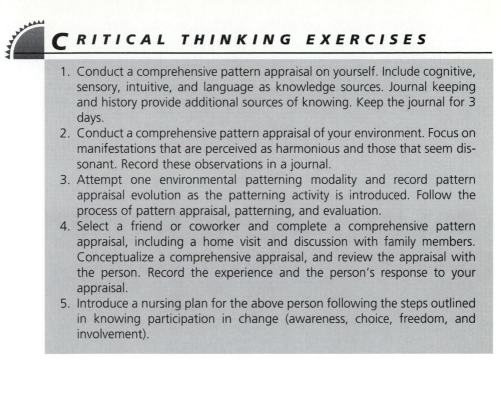

C R I T I C A L   T H I N K I N G   E X E R C I S E S

1. Conduct a comprehensive pattern appraisal on yourself. Include cognitive, sensory, intuitive, and language as knowledge sources. Journal keeping and history provide additional sources of knowing. Keep the journal for 3 days.
2. Conduct a comprehensive pattern appraisal of your environment. Focus on manifestations that are perceived as harmonious and those that seem dissonant. Record these observations in a journal.
3. Attempt one environmental patterning modality and record pattern appraisal evolution as the patterning activity is introduced. Follow the process of pattern appraisal, patterning, and evaluation.
4. Select a friend or coworker and complete a comprehensive pattern appraisal, including a home visit and discussion with family members. Conceptualize a comprehensive appraisal, and review the appraisal with the person. Record the experience and the person's response to your appraisal.
5. Introduce a nursing plan for the above person following the steps outlined in knowing participation in change (awareness, choice, freedom, and involvement).

References

Alligood, M. (1991). Testing Rogers' theory of accelerating change: The relationships among creativity, actualization, and empathy in persons 18-92 years of age. *Western Journal of Nursing Research, 13*(1), 84-96.

Alligood, M. (1994). Toward a unitary view of nursing practice. In M. Madrid and E. A. M. Barrett (Eds.), *Rogers' scientific art of nursing practice* (pp. 223-240). New York: National League for Nursing.

Barnum, B. (1990). *Nursing theory: Analysis, application, and evaluation* (3rd ed). Glenview, IL: Scott, Foresman/Little.

Barrett, E. (1986). Investigation of the principle of helicy: The relationship of human field motion and power. In V. Malinski (Ed.), *Explorations on Martha Rogers' science of unitary human beings,* (pp. 173-184). Norwalk, CT: Appleton-Century-Croft.

Barrett, E. (1990a). Health patterning with clients in a private practice environment. In E. Barrett (Ed.), *Visions of Rogers' science-based nursing* (pp. 105-115). New York: National League for Nursing.

Barrett, E. (1990b). Rogers' science-based nursing practice. In E. Barrett (Ed.), *Visions of Rogers' science-based nursing* (pp. 31-44). New York: National League for Nursing.

Bultemeier, K. (1993). *Photographic inquiry of the phenomenon premenstrual syndrome within the Rogerian-derived theory of perceived dissonance.* Unpublished doctoral dissertation, University of Tennessee, Knoxville.

Cowling, W. (1990). A template for unitary pattern–based nursing practice. In E. Barrett (Ed.), *Visions of Rogers' science-based nursing* (pp. 45-65). New York: National League for Nursing.

Daily, J., Maupin, J., Satterly, M., Schnell, D., & Wallace, T. (1989). Unitary human beings. In A. Marriner-Tomey (Ed.), *Nursing theorists and their work* (2nd ed., pp. 402-419). St. Louis: Mosby.

Kim, M. J., & Moritz, D. A. (1982). *Classification of nursing diagnosis: Proceedings of the third and fourth national conferences.* New York: McGraw-Hill.

Lutjens, L. R. J. (1991). *Martha Rogers: The science of unitary human beings.* Thousand Oaks, CA: Sage Publications.

Malinski, V. M. (1986a). Contemporary science and nursing: Parallels with Rogers. In V. Malinski (Ed.), *Explorations on Martha Rogers' science of unitary human beings* (pp. 15-23). Norwalk, CT: Appleton-Century-Croft.

Malinski, V. M. (1986b). Further ideas from Martha Rogers. In V. Malinski (Ed.), *Explorations on Martha Rogers' science of unitary human beings* (pp. 9-14). Norwalk, CT: Appleton-Century-Croft.

Malinski, V. M. (1986c). Nursing practice within the science of unitary human beings. In V. Malinski (Ed.), *Explorations on Martha Rogers' science of unitary human beings* (pp. 25-32). Norwalk, CT: Appleton-Century-Croft.

McDonald, S. F. (1986). The relationship between visible lightwaves and the experience of pain. In V. Malinski (Ed.), *Explorations on Martha Rogers' science of unitary human beings* (pp. 119-130). Norwalk, CT: Appleton-Century-Croft.

Parker, M. (1989). The theory of sentient evolution: A practice-level theory of sleeping, waking and beyond waking patterns based on the science of unitary human beings. *Rogerian Nursing Science News, 2*(1), 4-6.

Phillips, J. R. (1990). Changing human potentials and future visions of nursing: A human field image perspective. In E. A. Barrett (Ed.), *Visions of Rogers' science-based nursing* (pp. 13-25). New York: National League for Nursing.

Rogers, M. E. (1970). *An introduction to the theoretical basis of nursing.* Philadelphia: F. A. Davis.

Rogers, M. E. (1986). Science of unitary human beings. In V. Malinski (Ed.), *Explorations on Martha Rogers' science of unitary human beings* (pp. 3-8). Norwalk, CT: Appleton-Century-Crofts.

Rogers, M. E. (1990). Nursing: Science of unitary, irreducible, human beings: Update 1990. In E. Barrett (Ed.), *Visions of Rogers' science-based nursing* (pp. 5-11). New York: National League for Nursing.

Rogers, M. E. (1992). Nursing science and the space age. *Nursing Science Quarterly, 5,* 27-34.

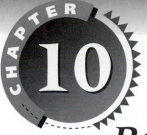

Roy's Adaptation Model in Nursing Practice

Kenneth D. Phillips

"The changing environment stimulates the person to make adaptive responses. For human beings, life is never the same. It is constantly changing and presenting new challenges. The person has the ability to make new responses to these changing conditions. As the environment changes, the person has the opportunity to continue to grow, to develop, and to enhance the meaning of life for everyone." (Andrews & Roy, 1991a)

Incessantly, human beings are besieged by a host of internal and external environmental stimuli. A stimulus is any entity that provokes a response (Andrews & Roy, 1991a). These environmental stimuli either threaten or enhance the individual's ability to adapt. As an example, loving, supportive behaviors from a parent enhance a child's ability to successfully adapt, whereas a hostile, abusive parent poses a threat to adaptation.

Nursing plays a vital role in assisting individuals sick or well to respond to a variety of new stressors, move toward optimal well-being, and improve the quality of their lives through adaptation. The Roy adaptation model (Roy & Andrews, 1991) provides an effective framework for addressing the adaptive needs of individuals and those of their families.

As noted in Chapter 1, nursing's most pressing question is, "What is the nature of the knowledge that is needed for the practice of nursing?" Nurses practicing within the Roy adaptation model seek (1) greater knowledge of factors that either promote or hinder adaptation, (2) better methods and tools for assessing adaptation level, (3) specific nursing interventions that either promote or hinder adaptation, and (4) effective methods for evaluating adaptation as an outcome of nursing care.

HISTORY AND BACKGROUND

Sister Callista Roy, a Sister of Saint Joseph of Carondelet, developed the Roy adaptation model (RAM) in 1964 in response to a challenge by her professor, Dorothy E. Johnson. Since that time, the RAM has experienced "being and becoming." The development of the model has been a dynamic process. The preliminary ideas of this conceptual framework were first published in an article entitled "Adaptation: A Conceptual Framework for Nursing" (Roy, 1970). The RAM continues to be refined. The Roy adaptation model is presented in its most complete and recent form in *The Roy Adaptation Model: The Definitive Statement* (Roy & Andrews, 1991). Many nurses in the United States, Canada, and worldwide practice nursing from the perspective of the RAM. The RAM has stimulated other scholars to publish books of their own about adaptation nursing (Randell, Poush Tedrow, & Van Landingham, 1982; Rambo, 1984; Welsh & Clochesy, 1990). The Roy adaptation model has been implemented in numerous hospitals and other healthcare settings. The RAM has been applied to diverse populations, adaptive needs, and developmental stages (Fawcett, 1995; Marriner-Tomey, 1994).

OVERVIEW OF ROY'S ADAPTATION MODEL

The RAM provides a useful framework for providing nursing care for persons in health and in acute, chronic, and terminal illness. The RAM views the person as an adaptive system in constant interaction with an internal and external environment. The environment is the source of a variety of stimuli that either threaten or promote the person's unique wholeness. The person's major task is to maintain integrity in face of these environmental stimuli. Roy, drawing on the work of Helson (1964), categorizes these stimuli as being either focal, contextual, or residual. The first type of stimulus, focal, is defined as the internal or external stimulus most immediately challenging the person's adaptation. The focal stimulus is the phenomenon that attracts one's attention. Contextual stimuli are all other stimuli existing in a situation that strengthen the effect of the focal stimulus. Residual stimuli are any other phenomena arising from a person's internal or external environment that may affect the focal stimulus but whose effects are unknown (Andrews & Roy, 1991a). The three types of stimuli act together and influence the adaptation level, which is a person's "ability to respond positively in a situation" (Andrews & Roy, 1991a, p. 10).

A person does not respond passively to environmental stimuli; the adaptation level is modulated by a person's coping mechanisms. Roy categorizes these coping mechanisms into either the regulator or the cognator subsystem. The coping mechanisms of the regulator subsystem occur through neural, chemical, and endocrine processes; the coping mechanisms of the cognator subsystem occur through cognitive-emotive processes (Andrews & Roy, 1991a).

Although direct observation of the processes of the regulator and cognator subsystems is not possible, Roy proposes that the behavioral responses of these two subsystems can be observed in any of the four adaptive modes: physiological, self-concept, role function, and interdependence adaptive modes. Roy and associates describe the function of the adaptive modes in the theory of the person as an adaptive system (Andrews & Roy, 1991a).

Roy's theory of the person as an adaptive system postulates that the four adaptive modes are interrelated through perception. Either an adaptive response or an ineffective response in one mode influences adaptation in the other modes.

The physiological adaptive mode refers to the "way a person responds as a physical being to stimuli from the environment" (Andrews & Roy, 1991a, p. 15). The five physiological needs of this mode are oxygenation, nutrition, elimination, activity and rest, and protection. Four complex processes that mediate the regulatory activity of this mode are senses, fluids and electrolytes, neurological function, and endocrine function. Physiological integrity is the adaptive response of this adaptive mode (Andrews & Roy, 1991c; Andrews & Roy, 1991a).

The self-concept adaptive mode refers to psychological and spiritual characteristics of the person (Andrews, 1991b; Andrews & Roy, 1991a). A person's self-concept consists of all the beliefs and feelings that one has formed about oneself. The self-concept is formed both from internal perceptions and from the perceptions of others. The self-concept changes over time and guides one's actions. The self-concept incorporates two components: the physical self and the personal self. The physical self incorporates body sensation and body image (Buck, 1991b). The personal self incorporates self-consistency, self-ideal, and moral-ethical-spiritual self (Buck, 1991a). Psychic integrity is the goal of the self-concept mode (Andrews, 1991b; Andrews & Roy, 1991a).

The interdependence adaptive mode refers to coping mechanisms that result in "the giving and receiving of love, respect, and value" (Andrews & Roy, 1991a, p. 17). In general, these contributive and receptive behaviors occur between the person and the most significant other or between the person and his/her support system. Affectional adequacy is the goal of the interdependence adaptive mode (Tedrow, 1991).

The role function adaptive mode refers to the primary, secondary, or tertiary roles the person performs in society. "A role, as the functioning unit of society, is defined as a set of expectations about how a person occupying one position behaves toward a person occupying another position" (Andrews & Roy, 1991a, p. 16). Social integrity is the goal of the role function mode (Andrews, 1991a; Nuwayhid, 1991).

Adaptive or ineffective responses result from these coping mechanisms. Adaptive responses promote the integrity of the person and the goals of adaptation, which are survival, growth, reproduction, and mastery (Andrews & Roy, 1991a). Ineffective responses neither promote integrity nor contribute to the goals of adaptation (Andrews & Roy, 1991a).

According to Roy, the major task of a person is to adapt to environmental stimuli in order to achieve survival, growth, development, and mastery. As described earlier, adaptation is accomplished through two main coping subsystems: regulator and cognator. Roy has not explicated the mechanisms of regulator and cognator because the mechanisms of regulator and cognator cannot be directly observed and remain largely unknown. However, the behaviors of regulator and cognator are manifested in the four adaptive modes (Roy, 1981), and the behaviors of regulator and cognator can be observed and measured in the four adaptive modes.

According to Roy, "health is a state and a process of being and becoming an integrated and whole person" (Andrews & Roy, 1991a, p. 19). Health is a reflection of how successfully an individual has adapted to environmental stimuli. The goal of nursing therefore is to help the person to achieve adaptation by helping the person to survive, grow, reproduce, and master. Adaptation leads to optimum health and well-being, to the highest quality of life possible, and to death with dignity (Andrews & Roy, 1991a). Adaptation enables the person to find meaning and purpose in life and to become an integrated whole.

CRITICAL THINKING IN NURSING PRACTICE WITH ROY'S MODEL

Nursing process is a goal-oriented, problem-solving approach to guide the provision of comprehensive, competent nursing care to a person or groups of persons. "Nursing process as described by Roy relates directly to the view of the person as an adaptive system" (Andrews & Roy, 1991b, p. 27). Roy has conceptualized the nursing process to be comprised of six simultaneous, ongoing, and dynamic steps. The steps of the nursing process are (1) assessment of behavior, (2) assessment of stimuli, (3) nursing diagnosis, (4) goal setting, (5) intervention, and (6) evaluation (Andrews & Roy, 1991b). Each of these phases of the nursing process is discussed within the RAM. The goal of nursing in the RAM is adaptation (Andrews & Roy, 1991a).

The nursing process alone is limited in promoting critical thinking; however, nursing theory serves as a guide for nursing care. Nursing theory directs the practitioner toward important aspects of assessing, planning, goal setting, implementation, and evaluation. Furthermore, practice within a model allows the practitioner to ignore irrelevant considerations and to selectively choose among a variety of nursing strategies. Another way of saying this is that nursing theory promotes critical thinking. Table 10-1 illustrates how the RAM guides the nurse through the critical thinking process.

Assessment of Behavior

According to Roy, behavior is an action or a reaction to a stimulus. A behavior is observable or nonobservable. An example of an observable behavior is pulse rate; a nonobservable behavior is a feeling experienced by the person and reported to the nurse. Exploration of behaviors manifested in the four adaptive modes allows the nurse to achieve an understanding of the current adaptation level and to plan interventions that will promote adaptation. At the beginning of the nurse-client relationship, a thorough assessment of behavior must be performed (Andrews & Roy, 1991b), and the assessment must be ongoing. Table 10-1 presents categories of behaviors that need to be assessed for each of the adaptive modes.

Assessment of Stimuli

According to Roy, a stimulus is any change in the internal or external environment that induces a response in the adaptive system. Stimuli that arise from the environment may be classified as focal, contextual, or residual. In this level of assessment, the nurse analyzes subjective and objective behaviors and looks more deeply for possible causes of a particular set of behaviors (Andrews & Roy, 1991b).

Nursing Diagnosis

A nurse's education and experience enable the nurse to make an expert judgment regarding healthcare and adaptive needs of the client. This judgment is expressed in a diagnostic statement that indicates an actual or a potential problem related to adaptation. The diagnostic statement specifies the behaviors that led to the diagnosis and a judgment regarding stimuli that threaten or promote adaptation (Andrews & Roy, 1991b). "Nursing diagnosis is defined in the RAM as a judgment process resulting in a statement conveying the person's adaptation status" (Andrews & Roy, 1991b, p. 37).

TABLE 10-1 Critical Thinking in the Roy Adaptation Model

Phases of Process	Physiological Adaptive Mode	Interdependence Adaptive Mode	Self-Concept Adaptive Mode	Role Function Adaptive Mode
Assessment of behavior	Oxygenation Nutrition Elimination Activity and rest Protection Senses Fluids and electrolytes Neurological function Endocrine function	Significant other Giving Receiving Support system Giving Receiving	Physical self Body sensation Body image Personal self Self-consistency Self-ideal Moral-ethical-spiritual self	Instrumental Primary role Secondary roles Tertiary roles Expressive Primary role Secondary roles Tertiary roles
Assessment of stimuli	Focal stimulus Contextual stimuli Residual stimuli	Focal stimulus Contextual stimuli Residual stimuli	Focal stimulus Contextual stimuli Residual stimuli	Focal stimulus Contextual stimuli Residual stimuli
Nursing diagnosis	Statement of behaviors with most relevant stimuli	Statement of behaviors with most relevant stimuli	Statement of behaviors with most relevant stimuli	Statement of behaviors with most relevant stimuli
Goal setting	Behavior Change expected Time frame	Behavior Change expected Time frame	Behavior Change expected Time frame	Behavior Change expected Time frame
Intervention	Management of stimuli Alter Increase Decrease Remove Maintain	Management of stimuli Alter Increase Decrease Remove Maintain	Management of stimuli Alter Increase Decrease Remove Maintain	Management of stimuli Alter Increase Decrease Remove Maintain
Evaluation	Observation of behaviors after interventions have been completed to see if goals have been obtained	Observation of behaviors after interventions have been completed to see if goals have been obtained	Observation of behaviors after interventions have been completed to see if goals have been obtained	Observation of behaviors after interventions have been completed to see if goals have been obtained

Goal Setting

Goal setting focuses on promoting adaptive behaviors. Together the nurse and the client agree on a statement about the desired outcome of nursing care. The outcome statement should (1) reflect a single adaptive behavior, (2) be realistic, and (3) be measurable. The goal statement should include the behavior to be changed, change expected, and time frame in which the change in behavior should occur (Andrews & Roy, 1991b).

Intervention

"Intervention focuses on the manner in which goals are attained" (Andrews & Roy, 1991b, p. 44). A nursing intervention is any action taken by a professional nurse that the nurse believes will promote adaptive behavior by a client. Nursing interventions arise from a solid knowledge base and are aimed at the focal stimulus whenever possible (Andrews & Roy, 1991b).

Evaluation

In the RAM, evaluation consists of one question: Has the person moved toward adaptation? Evaluation requires analysis and judgment to determine whether the behavioral changes desired in the goal statement have been achieved by the recipient of nursing care (Andrews & Roy, 1991b).

ASE HISTORY OF DEBBIE

Debbie is a 29-year-old woman who was recently admitted to the oncology nursing unit for evaluation after sensing pelvic "fullness" and noticing a watery, foul-smelling vaginal discharge. A Papanicolaou smear revealed a class V cervical cancer. She was found to have a stage II squamous cell carcinoma of the cervix and underwent a radical hysterectomy with bilateral salpingooophorectomy.

Her past health history revealed that physical examinations had been infrequent. She also reported that she has not performed breast self-examination. She is 5 feet 4 inches tall and weighs 89 pounds. Her usual weight is about 110 pounds. She has smoked approximately two packs of cigarettes a day for the past 16 years. She is gravida 2, para 2. Her first pregnancy was at age 16, and her second was at age 18. Since that time she has taken oral contraceptives on a regular basis.

Debbie completed the eighth grade. She is married and lives with her husband and two children in her mother's home, which she describes as less than sanitary. Her husband is unemployed. She describes him as emotionally distant and abusive at times.

She has done well following surgery except for being unable to completely empty her urinary bladder. She is having continued postoperative pain and nausea. It will be necessary for her to perform intermittent self-catheterization at home. Her home medications are (1) an antibiotic, (2) an analgesic as needed for pain, and (3) an antiemetic as needed for nausea. In addition, she will be receiving radiation therapy on an outpatient basis.

Debbie is extremely tearful. She expresses great concern over her future and the future of her two children. She believes that this illness is a punishment for her past life.

NURSING CARE OF DEBBIE WITH ROY'S MODEL
Physiological Adaptive Mode

Debbie's health problems are complex. It is impossible to develop interventions for all of her health problems within this chapter. Therefore only representative examples are presented.

Assessment of behavior. Postoperatively, Debbie has been unable to completely empty her urinary bladder. She states that she is "numb" and unable to tell when she needs to void. Catheterization for residual urine revealed that she was retaining 300 ml of urine after voiding. It will be necessary for her to perform intermittent self-catheterization at home. Unsanitary conditions at Debbie's home place her at high risk for developing a urinary tract infection. She states that she is "scared" about performing self-catheterization.

Assessment of stimuli. In this phase of the nursing process, the nurse searches for stimuli responsible for the observed behavior. After stimuli have been identified, they are classified as focal, contextual, or residual.

The focal stimulus for Debbie's urinary retention is the disease process. Contextual stimuli include tissue trauma resulting from surgery and radiation therapy. Debbie verified anxiety as a residual stimulus.

Infection is a potential problem. The focal stimulus is the need for intermittent self-catheterization. Contextual stimuli include altered skin integrity related to surgical incision, poor understanding of aseptic principles, and unsanitary conditions at Debbie's home.

Nursing diagnosis. From the assessment of behaviors and the assessment of stimuli, the following nursing diagnoses were made:
1. Altered elimination: urinary retention related to surgical trauma, radiation therapy, and anxiety
2. Potential for infection related to intermittent self-catheterization, altered skin integrity related to surgical incision, poor understanding of aseptic principles, and unsanitary conditions at Debbie's home

Goal setting. Goals were set mutually between the nurse and the client for each of the nursing diagnoses. The goals were:

1. Complete urinary elimination every 4 hours as evidenced by correct demonstration of the procedure for intermittent self-catheterization
2. Continued absence of signs of infection of the surgical incision and urinary tract

Implementation. To help Debbie attain these goals, the following nursing interventions were implemented:

1. *Altered elimination: urinary retention related to surgical trauma and radiation therapy*

Debbie was taught the importance of performing intermittent self-catheterization every 4 hours to prevent damage to the urinary bladder. She was taught to assess her abdomen for bladder distention and the proper procedure for intermittent self-catheterization. She was instructed to keep a record of the exact time and amount of voiding and catheterizations. In addition, Debbie was taught relaxation techniques to facilitate voiding so that it would not be necessary for her to catheterize herself as often.

2. *Potential for infection related to intermittent self-catheterization, altered skin integrity related to surgical incision, poor understanding of aseptic principles, and unsanitary conditions at Debbie's home*

Debbie was taught the importance of washing hands before touching the surgical incision or doing incision care. The procedure for incision care was demonstrated by the nursing staff, and Debbie was asked to perform a return demonstration. After the intermittent self-catheterization procedure was explained and demonstrated, Debbie was asked to perform a return demonstration.

Evaluation. Evaluation of Debbie's adaptive level was performed each shift. Significant findings included:

1. It will be necessary for her to perform intermittent self-catheterization at home. Debbie was able to state the importance of performing intermittent self-catheterization on a regular basis. She performed a return demonstration of intermittent self-catheterization before discharge, and she was able to adequately adhere to aseptic principles during the procedure. She accurately recorded the times and amount for each voiding and catheterization.
2. Debbie was able to list the signs and symptoms of a wound and a urinary tract infection and to state appropriate steps to take if symptoms occur (i.e., notify physician or nurse practitioner). She was able to discuss the importance of maintaining adequate oral fluid intake. Debbie was given a thermometer and instructed in its use. She correctly demonstrated taking a temperature.

Interdependence Adaptive Mode
Assessment of behavior

Significant other. Debbie's most significant other is her husband. She describes her husband as emotionally distant and abusive at times. He has been at the bedside since Debbie was admitted to the hospital. He appears worried. In addition to these findings, it would be important to determine how Debbie and her husband give and receive love, value, and respect and how they express nurturing and caring behaviors to each other.

Support system. Debbie's support system includes her mother and her two children. Debbie and her family live in her mother's home. It is important to know how Debbie and her support system give and receive love, value, and respect and how they express nurturing and caring behaviors to each other.

Assessment of stimuli. Assessment of stimuli within the interdependence adaptive mode reveals that Debbie's relationship needs with her husband are not being met. It is encouraging that her husband is displaying nurturing, caring behaviors while Debbie is in the hospital. Further evaluation of Debbie's self-esteem would be warranted. Debbie and her husband were married at an early age. Their knowledge regarding building friendships and relationships may be limited. It would be important to assess modes of communication as well. The developmental stage for Debbie and her husband is that of young adults. In this stage, the individual becomes independent and establishes his/her own family. Debbie and her family live with her mother. This may be creating a stress on interdependence. Debbie acknowledges that she and her husband have very little time alone.

The focal stimulus in the interdependence adaptive mode is an emotionally distant relationship with her husband. Contextual stimuli are (1) Debbie and her husband were married at an early age following an unplanned pregnancy, (2) they exhibit ineffective communication skills, (3) they live with her mother, and (4) they have very little time alone.

Nursing diagnosis. The following nursing diagnoses of interdependence adaptive needs were made:
1. Affectional inadequacy related to emotionally distant relationship, marriage at an early age following an unplanned pregnancy, ineffective communication skills, living with a parent, and having very little time alone
2. Potential change in support system dynamics related to potential role changes and changes in health status

Goal setting. To help Debbie with these adaptive needs, the following goals were agreed on:
1. Increased affectional adequacy between Debbie and her husband by discharge as manifested by verbalization of and a need for increased communication between Debbie and her husband
2. Support system dynamics will remain stable during Debbie's recovery period

Implementation. To help Debbie attain these goals, the following nursing interventions were implemented:
1. *Affectional inadequacy related to emotionally distant relationship, marriage at an early age following an unplanned pregnancy, ineffective communication skills, living with a parent, and having very little time alone*

Assessment of interdependence was begun while performing other routine care. Debbie was asked questions like: (1) Can you tell me about your relationship? (2) Do you consider it a "good" relationship? (3) What do you think would make a good relationship? (4) How does your husband express to you that he loves you? (5) How do you express to your husband that you love him? (6) How do you and your husband talk about things important to you?

Debbie's husband has been with her much of the time she has been hospitalized, and he seemed worried. Her husband was encouraged to do back massage when Debbie was experiencing pain or to just hold her hand when she became tearful.
2. *Potential change in support system dynamics related to potential role changes and changes in health status*

With Debbie's permission, time was allocated to discuss important aspects of relationship building. Both Debbie and her husband were agreeable. Professional family counseling services were obtained through the parish nursing ministry of the hospital for Debbie's family.

Evaluation. Debbie was pleased that her husband was talking to her more and enjoyed the caring behaviors in which he was participating. They began their counseling sessions before Debbie's discharge. They both resolved to spend more time alone. They both felt the counseling was worthwhile and wanted to continue after discharge.

Self-Concept Adaptive Mode

Assessment of behavior. Debbie is extremely tearful. She expresses great concern over her future and the future of her children. Exploration of Debbie's tearfulness revealed that Debbie was afraid of dying. She believes that this illness is a punishment for her past behavior. Debbie and her husband were married at a very young age after Debbie became pregnant with their first child.

Debbie has not asked the nurse any questions about sexuality. Her hesitancy to introduce the subject may be related to her cultural background. In this case the nurse introduces the topic. Salient findings here are (1) Debbie recently learned of a diagnosis of cervical cancer; (2) she has undergone a recent radical hysterectomy; (3) she is receiving radiation therapy in the hospital, and the need for this therapy will continue at home; (4) Debbie has a lack of information about the impact of cervical cancer, radical hysterectomy, and chemotherapy on sexuality; and (5) Debbie has unresolved guilt related to unplanned premarital pregnancy.

Assessment of stimuli. Debbie is a young adult, she is married, and she has two young children. Debbie has an eighth grade education. She is in an emotionally distant, sometimes abusive relationship. Being diagnosed with cervical cancer at an early age has resulted in a maturational crisis for Debbie. This is complicated by the fact that several of her relatives have died of cancer. It is important for the nurse to assess coping strategies. One coping strategy that is mentioned is that Debbie is frequently tearful.

Nursing diagnosis. The following nursing diagnoses were made:
1. Fear and anxiety of dying related to medical diagnosis and witnessing other family members' deaths as a result of cancer
2. Spiritual distress related to severe life-threatening illness and unresolved guilt related to unplanned premarital pregnancy
3. Sexual dysfunction related to the disease process, recent radical hysterectomy, need for radiation therapy at home, loss of childbearing capacity, weakness, fatigue, pain, anxiety, hormonal changes, and a lack of information about the impact of cervical cancer, radical hysterectomy, and chemotherapy on sexuality
4. Grieving related to body image disturbance, loss of self-ideal, changes in roles, and potential for premature death

Goal setting. To help Debbie achieve adaptation in the interdependence adaptive mode, the following goals were mutually set:
1. Decreased fear and anxiety of dying as evidenced by less tearfulness, relaxed facial expression, relaxed body movements, verbalization of new coping strategies, and fewer verbalizations of fear and anxiety
2. Decreased spiritual distress as evidenced by verbalization of positive feelings about self, verbalization about the value and meaning of her life, and less tearfulness

3. Resumed sexual relationship that is satisfying to both partners as evidenced by verbalization of self as sexually capable and acceptable, verbalization of alternative methods of sexual expression during the first 6 weeks following surgery, and verbalization of when to be able to resume vaginal intercourse
4. Progression through the grieving process as evidenced by verbalization of feelings regarding body image, self-ideal, changes in roles, and potential for premature death

Implementation. The following nursing interventions were implemented to help achieve these goals in the self-concept adaptive mode:
1. *Fear and anxiety of dying related to medical diagnosis and witnessing other family members' deaths as a result of cancer*

Although Debbie's prognosis appeared good, she remained fearful of dying. Time was taken to sit with Debbie, make eye contact, and actively listen to her, especially when she began crying.

Debbie was asked to share an extremely difficult experience she had encountered in the past. She was asked how she coped with that experience. Once her present coping strategies were assessed, new coping strategies were suggested.

She was encouraged to express her feelings openly. After allowing Debbie adequate time to express her feelings, truthful and realistic hope based on Debbie's medical history was offered. A cancer support group met each Tuesday in the hospital where Debbie was a patient. Debbie was given a schedule of the meeting times and topics. She and her husband were encouraged to attend the cancer support group meetings.

2. *Spiritual distress related to severe life-threatening illness and perception of moral-ethical-spiritual self*

Debbie was encouraged to express her feelings openly about her illness. It was suggested that times of illness are good times to renew spiritual ties. Debbie was supported in positive aspects of her life (e.g., being a good mother). At Debbie's request, the parish nursing ministry was consulted, and a chaplain was asked to visit Debbie.

3. *Sexual dysfunction related to the disease process, recent radical hysterectomy, need for radiation therapy at home, loss of childbearing capacity, weakness, fatigue, pain, anxiety, hormonal changes, and a lack of information about the impact of cervical cancer, radical hysterectomy, and chemotherapy on sexuality*

A complete sexual assessment was conducted to evaluate the perceived adequacy of Debbie's sexual relationship and to elicit concerns or issues about sexuality before her diagnosis with cervical cancer. Private conversation was initiated with Debbie to gain an understanding of her sexual concerns resulting from her therapy and her beliefs about the effect of radical hysterectomy in regard to sexual functioning. Debbie was instructed regarding possible changes in sexual functioning such as a temporary loss of vaginal sensation for up to several months, vaginal dryness, and dyspareunia resulting from vaginal dryness. Since vaginal intercourse would not be possible for up to 6 weeks, alternate forms of sexual expression were discussed. To facilitate communication and sexual expression between Debbie and her husband, long periods of uninterrupted privacy were provided.

4. *Grieving related to body image disturbance, loss of self-ideal, changes in roles, and potential for premature death*

Debbie's perceptions regarding the impact of the diagnosis of cervical cancer on her body image, self-ideal, roles, and her future were explored. Debbie was encouraged to verbally acknowledge the losses that she was experiencing. Debbie was observed to determine which stage of the grief process she was currently experiencing (denial, anger, bargaining, depression, or acceptance) (Kubler-Ross, 1969). The grieving process was explained to Debbie and to her family, and they were assured that grieving is a normal process. Family members were encouraged to allow Debbie to cry when she needed to cry and to talk about her fears and feelings of grief. The nursing staff offered realistic reassurance about Debbie's prognosis. Debbie was encouraged to attend the cancer support group so that she could talk to others who better understood her grief.

Evaluation. Debbie's behavior changed before discharge. At the cancer support group, Debbie met Marie, a survivor of cervical cancer. After meeting Marie, Debbie became more hopeful that she could conquer cancer. Less tearful, Debbie appeared more relaxed. Debbie verbalized a good understanding of sexual changes that would occur and ways to help her adapt to these changes.

Role Function Adaptive Mode

Assessment of behavior. Assessment in the role function adaptive mode requires the nurse to identify primary, secondary, and tertiary roles. When these roles have been identified, the nurse looks for instrumental and expressive behaviors related to each of these roles. An instrumental behavior is an actual physical act performed by the individual that helps achieve the goal of mastery of a primary, secondary, or tertiary role. An expressive behavior is the attitude or feeling a person holds about a primary, secondary, or tertiary role.

Assessment of behaviors in the role function adaptive mode revealed that Debbie loves her husband very much and want things to be better for them. She is a conscientious mother. She is a dutiful daughter who assists her mother as needed. She enjoys helping elders in her community because it makes her feel good to help others when they need it. She has been diagnosed with cervical cancer, undergone radical hysterectomy, and is being treated with radiation therapy.

Assessment of stimuli. The focal stimulus in the role function adaptive mode is the fear of not being able to care for herself or her children in the future. Contextual stimuli include severe illness, radiation therapy, weakness, fatigue, and increased dependency on others.

Nursing diagnosis. The following nursing diagnoses were made:
1. Ineffective primary role transition related to severe illness, radiation therapy, weakness, fatigue, and increased dependency on others
2. Ineffective secondary role transition related to fear of not being able to care for herself or her children in the future

Goal setting. To help Debbie achieve adaptation in the role function adaptive mode, the following goals were mutually set:
1. Effective primary role transition as manifested by less weakness, less fatigue, willingness to allow others to help her when she needs assistance, and desire to resume self-care activities as she becomes able
2. Effective secondary role transition as manifested by fewer verbalizations of anxiety over her ability to care for herself and her children in the future

Implementation. The following nursing interventions were implemented to help achieve these goals in the role function adaptive mode:
1. *Ineffective primary role transition related to severe illness, radiation therapy, weakness, fatigue, and increased dependency on others*

Debbie was monitored for factors that would hinder her from performing self-care activities. A daily routine was established that incorporated periods of activity and periods of rest. Measures were implemented to promote rest (e.g., activity restrictions, minimal noise, restricted visitation, a morning and afternoon nap time, assistance with personal care, needed items close to her bed, back massage, progressive relaxation, guided imagery, and soft music). However, maximum independence was encouraged. Family members were instructed regarding the importance of maintaining independence. She was given positive reinforcement for successful accomplishment of self-care behaviors.

Debbie was praised for her performance of her primary, secondary, and tertiary roles. Resumption of these roles were discussed with Debbie. Debbie was asked to identify her support system. She felt that she had adequate support at home with performing her roles. She was encouraged to rely on her support system for help when needed in maintaining these roles.

2. *Ineffective secondary role transition related to fear of not being able to care for herself or her children in the future*

A thorough assessment was performed to gain an understanding of Debbie's fears and misconceptions about the effects of cancer, radical hysterectomy, and radiation therapy on bodily functioning, her lifestyle, and her ability to perform roles. Debbie verbalized a fear of dying and leaving her children. Interventions to instill hope were implemented. For instance, Debbie was given realistic assurance about her expected prognosis.

Evaluation. Debbie's husband was exhibiting supportive behaviors in the hospital. Debbie's mother was at home to help Debbie when she arrived. As Debbie's energy level was increased, she became less anxious over her future. Before discharge, Debbie became increasingly anxious to return home to her children.

ASE HISTORY OF BOBBY

Bobby is a 27-year-old white, homosexual man. After experiencing severe diarrhea and pronounced weight loss, he scheduled an appointment with his family physician. Both enzyme-linked immunoassay (ELISA) and Western blot tests indicated that Bobby was infected with HIV.

Bobby lost 31 pounds over the last 6 weeks. His weight loss has been rapid and unintentional. He complains of mouth soreness, dysphagia, anorexia, and that foods have less taste than usual. White patches are observed over the tongue, buccal mucosa, and palate. He reports poor nutritional habits.

Bobby began having infrequent episodes of diarrhea about 2 months ago. Both the frequency and amount of watery diarrhea have increased over time. This has led to a fluid volume deficit. A stool culture revealed the presence of *Cryptosporidium muris*.

Bobby's family consists of his partner of 5 years, mother, father, and sister. By his acknowledgment, Bobby's most emotionally intimate relationship is with his sister. He states that he can share his deepest fears, thoughts, and wishes with her. Bobby relates well to his sister, her husband, and his two teenage nephews. She visits him daily and brings food and fresh flowers from the garden that they had planted together. She speaks gently to him and holds his hand when he is upset.

Bobby lives with his partner, Matt, in a small house on property that is owned by his sister and her husband. Matt has shown great concern about Bobby's health. Matt continues to work as a teacher and provides both emotional and financial support for Bobby. Matt is seronegative for HIV, and fear of contagion is a source of anxiety for both Bobby and Matt.

Bobby has a number of gay friends. None of his gay friends has visited. Bobby does not call his friends on the telephone because he does not "want to discuss AIDS with them." He communicates minimally with family and friends. Bobby states that he has had lots of friends in the past and that he has done many things for them. He asks, "Where are they when I need them?" He complains of being lonely much of the time.

Bobby's parents live in another city, and he has had a distant relationship with them for the past 10 years. His father is a minister in a fundamentalist, Protestant denomination. Bobby has been unable to discuss being gay with his parents because he knows they would disapprove. He fears being abandoned by his parents.

Bobby's primary role is that of a young adult. Bobby's secondary roles include partner, son, brother, brother-in-law, uncle, and friend. Bobby has always assumed the "caretaker" role where Matt is concerned. He is sad that Matt is now having to do so many things for him. Bobby's sister has stated that she is not afraid, but she expresses some concern that her children might not be careful enough.

Bobby is a paramedic. He has enjoyed working as a paramedic for the past 8 years. He is questioning whether he will be able to work in this occupation in the future. Bobby's physician recommended to him that he resign his job. He talks about "all the adjustments" that he will have to make in his life. Bobby expresses guilt about all the responsibility that his illness has placed on Matt and other members of his family.

Bobby has always been concerned with his appearance. He has remained physically fit. He dresses neatly, but now his clothing is fitting more loosely. Bobby expresses concern about his "deteriorating" physical appearance and his lack of energy. Matt reports that he lies in bed most of the time, sighs often, and begins crying frequently. He asks, "Why is this happening to me? I don't deserve this. I am a good person." Things that he indicates make him feel better about himself are his job, regular physical workouts, and his friends.

NURSING CARE OF BOBBY WITH ROY'S MODEL
Physiological Adaptive Mode

Assessment of behavior. Bobby is a cachectic 27-year-old man. He has lost 31 pounds over the last 6 weeks. His weight loss has been rapid and unintentional. He complains of mouth soreness, dysphagia, anorexia, and that foods have less taste than usual. White patches are observed over the tongue, buccal mucosa, and palate. He reports poor nutritional habits.

Assessment of stimuli. It was determined by assessment of stimuli that the focal stimulus for Bobby's weight loss was increased metabolic demands as a result of HIV infection. Contextual stimuli contributing to the weight loss were mouth soreness, difficulty chewing, difficulty swallowing, decreased taste of foods, and poor dietary choices (Flaskerud & Ungvarski, 1995).

Nursing diagnosis. The following nursing diagnosis was made in the physiological adaptive mode:

1. Alterations in nutrition: less than body requirements related to increased metabolic demands as the result of infection, mouth soreness, difficulty chewing, difficulty swallowing, and decreased taste of foods

Goal setting. The following goal was mutually established:
1. Improved nutritional status as evidenced by (a) no further weight loss during the next week and (b) improved appetite within 24 hours

Implementation. So that Bobby could achieve his goal for improved nutritional status, the following interventions were implemented:
1. *Alterations in nutrition: less than body requirements related to increased metabolic demands as the result of infection, mouth soreness, difficulty chewing, difficulty swallowing, and decreased taste of foods*

Bobby was given verbal and written instructions on methods to increase his dietary intake of protein, carbohydrates, fats, and total calories. Bobby was advised to drink three cans of liquid nutritional supplements (e.g., Ensure, Advera) per day. A daily vitamin and a mineral supplement were recommended. Arrangements were made for a hot lunch to be delivered each day by the local AIDS support group. As suggested, Bobby began eating six small meals each day. Bobby's weight was measured each week (Task Force on Nutrition Support in AIDS, 1989).

Evaluation. Bobby's appetite was slowly improving. He gained 1 lb during the next week. Bobby reported less pain when chewing and swallowing. Bobby's intake and output averaged approximately 2400 ml per day during the next 3 days.

Interdependence Adaptive Mode

Assessment of behavior. Bobby's family consists of his partner, sister, brother-in-law, nephews, mother, and father. He has a good relationship with his partner, but his most emotionally intimate relationship is with his sister. He has a number of gay friends, but none of them has visited. He does not call his friends. Bobby has been unable to share with his parents that he is gay or that he has HIV infection.

Assessment of stimuli. Bobby is estranged from his parents and his gay friends. The focal stimulus for this estrangement is HIV infection. The contextual stimuli are related to his self-concept. These contextual stimuli are internalized stigma of AIDS (Phillips, 1994), which prevents Bobby from contacting his gay friends, and internalized homophobia (Nungesser, 1978, 1979, 1983), which prevents communication between Bobby and his parents.

Nursing diagnosis. The following nursing diagnosis of the interdependent adaptive needs was made:

1. Alienation related to HIV infection, internalized stigma of AIDS, and internalized homophobia

Goal setting. To help Bobby experience a decreased sense of alienation, the following goals were mutually set:

1. Maintenance of relationships with his family and friends
2. Talking to friends on the telephone by the end of the week
3. Verbalization of decreased feeling of loneliness
4. Participation in a diversional activity of his choice
5. Exploration of the possibility of attending the local AIDS support group next week

Implementation. To help Bobby attain these goals, the following nursing interventions were implemented:

1. *Alienation related to HIV infection, internalized stigma of AIDS, internalized homophobia*

Bobby was assessed regularly for signs of increasing social isolation such as decreased communication with family and friends. Bobby was encouraged to express his feelings of loneliness freely and openly. Because Bobby had a fear of contracting an infection from others, it was explained that contact with healthy adults was not a source of infection for him. Knowing Bobby's relationship with Matt, Matt was included in discussions regarding Bobby's care. Bobby was urged to contact his friends by telephone. Bobby's gift at watercolor painting was obvious from his artwork displayed in his home, and he was encouraged to continue this hobby. Since Bobby was constantly concerned about telling his parents about his illness, role playing was suggested. The nurse played the role of Bobby's father and asked him to tell whatever he would like for his father to know. Bobby was asked to think about where he would like to be when he tells his parents about his HIV infection and whom he would like to be with him for support when he tells his parents. He was encouraged to ask others in the AIDS support group how they handled this situation.

Evaluation. Bobby continued to be receptive to giving and receiving love and support from Matt and his sister. He remained hesitant to talk to his friends on the telephone. He spent a great deal of time watching the television. He felt that his energy level was too low for painting. At Bobby's request, a visitor from the local AIDS support group came to visit Bobby. Bobby stated later that he really enjoyed that visit. He indicated to the visitor that he would like to attend the support group sessions when he is discharged from the hospital. Bobby's parents came to visit him as soon as they heard that he was in the hospital. In the next few hours, they learned both that Bobby had AIDS and that he was gay. They had suspected for many years that Bobby was gay. Bobby's father assured him that God loves him, that God would forgive him, that God would change him.

Self-Concept Adaptive Mode

Assessment of behavior. Bobby has not shared with his parents that he is gay or that he has HIV infection. He is concerned about his "deteriorating" physical appearance and his lack of energy. He lies in the bed most of the time, sighs often, and begins crying frequently. He asks, "Why is this happening to me? I don't deserve this. I am a good person."

Assessment of stimuli. Bobby comes from a devoutly religious family and a religion that teaches that homosexuality is morally wrong. Bobby has found it difficult to tell his family that he is gay and has postponed telling them that he has HIV infection. The focal stimulus is HIV infection. Contextual stimuli are internalized stigma of AIDS (Phillips, 1994) and internalized homophobia (Nungesser, 1978, 1979, 1983). A residual stimulus was fear of losing his parents' support.

Nursing diagnosis. The following nursing diagnoses of self-concept adaptive needs were made:
1. Grief related to changes in current and anticipated physical appearance, lifestyle, sexual dysfunction, anticipated loss of health status, and probable impending death
2. Spiritual distress related to severe, life-threatening illness and alternative lifestyle
3. Sexual dysfunction related to fear of transmitting HIV infection

Goal setting. To help Bobby meet self-concept adaptive needs, the following goals were mutually set:
1. A resolution of grief as manifested by verbalization of moving through the grief process
2. Increased experience of spirituality as manifested by verbalization of meaning and purpose of life and verbalization of connectedness with self, others, and God
3. Continuation of a mutually satisfying sexual relationship between Bobby and Matt and identification of methods to prevent the transmission of HIV

Implementation. To help Bobby achieve these goals, the following interventions were employed:

1. *Grief related to changes in current and anticipated physical appearance, lifestyle, sexual dysfunction, anticipated loss of health status, and probable impending death*

An assessment of Bobby's perception of the impact of AIDS on his physical appearance, sexual functioning, health status, and future was performed. Active listening skills and therapeutic communication techniques were used to assist Bobby in verbalizing his feelings and acknowledging losses he was experiencing. Bobby was asked to express a stressful event in the past and to discuss coping mechanisms that helped him get through that stressful event. Bobby and his partner had a good understanding of the stages of the normal grieving process. His behavior was observed to determine his current stage of the grieving process. Family members were encouraged to allow him to express his feelings freely.

2. *Spiritual distress related to severe, life-threatening illness and alternative lifestyle*

Fear is a significant component of spiritual distress. Fear may be related to rejection and separation from others related to the diagnosis of AIDS or a feeling of separation from God (Coward & Lewis, 1993). Bobby was encouraged to strengthen connections with old friends and to develop connections with new friends. Bobby was encouraged to experience connectedness with the universe through field trips, meditation, and guided imagery. Bobby's beliefs about a higher power were assessed. Bobby was encouraged to continue his belief in a loving God. Bobby was encouraged to spend time in meditation and prayer to discover more of this love.

Fear of the dying process may contribute to spiritual distress (Coward & Lewis, 1993). Bobby was encouraged to express his fears related to the dying process. Participation in the AIDS support group was recommended.

The fear of dying without making a lasting contribution to society is another element of spiritual distress (Coward & Lewis, 1993). When Bobby verbalized this fear, he was encouraged to look for ways to leave a lasting legacy. Bobby was encouraged to talk about his past events, interests, hobbies, occupation, and feelings. Bobby was prompted to focus on positive aspects of his life rather than negative ones.

Bobby was encouraged to seek out new challenges and to do some of the things that he had always wanted to do (Coward & Lewis, 1993). Bobby's watercolor painting became an outlet for his feelings. As Bobby's health improved, he began a small gardening business. During the Christmas shopping season, he opened a shop in the shopping mall where he sold his bonsai creations.

Hope and spirituality are intertwined. Bobby's sense of hope was assessed. He continued to be hopeful that a cure would be found. That hope was supported. However, his hope was tied to the present rather than to the future. He was encouraged to engage in self-care behaviors that would help him remain healthy. As the disease progressed, he was supported in his acceptance of his prognosis.

3. *Sexual dysfunction related to fear of transmitting HIV infection*

Active listening and therapeutic communication techniques were employed to facilitate expression of fears. Communication between Bobby and Matt was encouraged. Bobby and Matt were given factual information regarding HIV transmission. Instructions for the proper use of a latex condom containing nonoxynol 9 during insertive sexual techniques were given. Bobby was instructed to wash his hands after toileting and after contact with body fluids such as semen, mucus, or blood. Matt was instructed to avoid contact with body fluids such as semen, mucus, or blood. Bobby and Matt were instructed to avoid sharing eating utensils, towels, wash cloths, toothbrushes, razors, nail clippers, and sexual devices. Alternative forms of noninsertive sexual practices were discussed. Bobby and Matt were encouraged to attend the AIDS support group meetings to learn more about prevention.

Evaluation. Bobby moved appropriately through the stages of grief. Although he has accepted the fact that his death is probably imminent, he continues to experience the fullness of life.

Bobby demonstrated increased spirituality. He has become very active and serves as a deacon in a church where he is readily accepted. He derives pleasure from helping others who have HIV infection. He has started two small businesses since he became ill.

Bobby and Matt are able to verbalize understanding of principles to prevent HIV transmission. Bobby and Matt report a mutually satisfying sexual relationship.

Role Function Adaptive Mode

Assessment of behavior. Bobby's primary role is that of a young adult. His secondary roles include partner, son, brother, brother-in-law, uncle, and friend. He is a paramedic. His physician has recommended that he resign from his job. Bobby talks about "all the adjustments" he will have to make in his life.

Assessment of stimuli. The focal stimulus in this adaptive mode is HIV infection. Contextual stimuli include the potential loss of employment and income and feeling guilty about the hardship his illness is causing others.

Nursing diagnosis. In nursing, the family is viewed as the client. HIV infection will greatly impact the lives of all those in Bobby's family. The following nursing diagnosis was made:

1. Ineffective role transition related to loss of employment, guilt about the responsibility his illness has placed on his family members, and the fear that he is not going to be able to "make it" financially

Goal setting. The following goals were mutually set:
1. Bobby: effective primary role transition as evidenced by increased verbalization of his feelings about HIV infection and impending loss of independence
2. Bobby: effective secondary role transition as evidenced by increased verbalization of his feelings regarding resignation from his job, increased verbalization of his feelings about the many changes in secondary roles that he is encountering, and by assumption of responsibility for applying for benefits to which he is entitled
3. Bobby's sister: effective secondary role transition as evidenced by verbalization of less anxiety and fear about her children becoming infected with HIV
4. Bobby's family members: effective secondary role transition as evidenced by participating in support group meetings, increased verbalization of their feelings regarding Bobby's illness, and taking time for personal and family needs

Implementation. Bobby was encouraged to freely express his feelings regarding the many changes in his life. Bobby was encouraged to attend the AIDS support group meetings. Time was allocated to just sit and talk with Bobby. Therapeutic communication techniques were used to facilitate Bobby's expression of his feelings.

Bobby's change in employment status was a major concern for Bobby. Bobby was encouraged to explore his feelings about resigning from his job. Work was begun to help Bobby find alternative sources of income. Supplemental Security Income (SSI) forms were obtained. Bobby and Matt were encouraged to complete the forms together.

By revealing that she was concerned that her children might become infected with HIV, Bobby's sister was sharing her fear of infection as well. Time was set aside for discussing these fears. Role modeling by the nurse was an important intervention that was used. At Bobby's request, a session was arranged with his sister's family to discuss infection control principles. Age-appropriate written information about infection control principles was given to each of the family members. Bobby's sister, her husband, and Matt were encouraged to attend AIDS caregivers support group meetings.

HIV infection places enormous responsibilities on families. Family members were encouraged to maintain open communication and to share feelings with each other. Family members were encouraged to take time for themselves and for family activities.

Evaluation. Bobby increasingly verbalized his feelings and his fears. By attending support groups meetings, Bobby became aware of many services that were available to him in the community. He and Matt took an active role in "learning the system" about procuring resources from government agencies that Bobby needed. After Bobby resigned his job, he became a volunteer for the AIDS support group. After receiving information about how HIV is transmitted, Bobby's sister became less fearful. Bobby was able to maintain close relationships with his nephews. Many extra responsibilities were imposed on the family by Bobby's illness. Bobby's sister rearranged her busy schedule so that she could continue to help Bobby and still spend time with her family.

CRITICAL THINKING EXERCISES

Critical thinking using Roy's model moves the nurse beyond the assessment phase of the nursing process to (1) identifying stimuli that cause problems in adaptation, (2) making appropriate nursing diagnoses, (3) establishing meaningful goals, (4) applying innovative nursing interventions, and (5) evaluating the effectiveness of nursing care in moving the client toward adaptation. The following exercises demonstrate critical thinking from the perspective of the RAM.

1. In the case of Bobby under the role function adaptive mode, identify which goal is being met in the discussion of implementation on p. 197.
2. You have just been notified that you have won $30,000,000 in the Virginia State Lottery. Undoubtedly, this would lead to a significant change in your adaptive level. Using Roy's principles of a two-level assessment (assessment of behaviors and assessment of stimuli):
   a. List possible behaviors for each of the four adaptive modes.
   b. Identify focal, contextual, and residual stimuli for each of the four adaptive modes.
3. Your closest friend has just been diagnosed with breast cancer. She has undergone a radical mastectomy. She is receiving chemotherapy. She has just learned that the condition is terminal. She is single, and she has a daughter who is 6 years old.
   a. What would be her adaptive needs in the physiological adaptive mode? What interventions would you provide?
   b. What would be her adaptive needs in the self-concept adaptive mode? What interventions would you provide?
   c. What would be her adaptive needs in the interdependence adaptive mode? What interventions would you provide?
   d. What would be her adaptive needs in the role function adaptive mode? What interventions would you provide?

Continued.

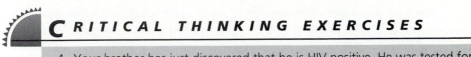

CRITICAL THINKING EXERCISES

4. Your brother has just discovered that he is HIV positive. He was tested for HIV after his girlfriend told him that she was seropositive. Because you are a nurse, you are the first member of his family whom he has told.
   a. What would be his adaptive needs in the physiological adaptive mode? What interventions would you provide?
   b. What would be his adaptive needs in the self-concept adaptive mode? What interventions would you provide?
   c. What would be his adaptive needs in the interdependence adaptive mode? What interventions would you provide?
   d. What would be his adaptive needs in the role function adaptive mode? What interventions would you provide?

References

Andrews, H. A. (1991a). Overview of the role function mode. In Sr. C. Roy & H. A. Andrews (Eds.), *The Roy adaptation model: The definitive statement* (pp. 347-361). Norwalk, CT: Appleton & Lange.

Andrews, H. A. (1991b). Overview of the self-concept mode. In Sr. C. Roy & H. A. Andrews (Eds.), *The Roy adaptation model: The definitive statement* (pp. 269-279). Norwalk, CT: Appleton & Lange.

Andrews, H. A., & Roy, Sr. C. (1991a). Essentials of the Roy adaptation model. In Sr. C. Roy & H. A. Andrews (Eds.), *The Roy adaptation model: The definitive statement* (pp. 2-25). Norwalk, CT: Appleton & Lange.

Andrews, H. A., & Roy, Sr. C. (1991b). The nursing process according to the Roy adaptation model. In Sr. C. Roy & H. A. Andrews (Eds.), *The Roy adaptation model: The definitive statement* (pp. 27-54). Norwalk, CT: Appleton & Lange.

Andrews, H. A., & Roy, Sr. C. (1991c). Overview of the physiological adaptive mode. In Sr. C. Roy & H. A. Andrews (Eds.), *The Roy adaptation model: The definitive statement* (pp. 57-66). Norwalk, CT: Appleton & Lange.

Buck, M. H. (1991a). The personal self. In Sr. C. Roy & H. A. Andrews (Eds.), *The Roy adaptation model: The definitive statement* (pp. 311-335). Norwalk, CT: Appleton & Lange.

Buck, M. H. (1991b). The physical self. In Sr. C. Roy & H. A. Andrews (Eds.), *The Roy adaptation model: The definitive statement* (pp. 281-310). Norwalk, CT: Appleton & Lange.

Coward, D. D., & Lewis, F. M. (1993). The lived experience of self-transcendence in gay men with AIDS. *Oncology Nursing Forum, (20)*9, 1363-1368.

Fawcett, J. (1995). *Analysis and evaluation of conceptual models of nursing* (3rd ed.). Philadelphia: F. A. Davis.

Flaskerud, J. H., & Ungvarski, P. J. (1995). *HIV/AIDS: A guide to nursing care* (3rd ed.). Philadelphia: W. B. Saunders.

Helson, H. (1964). *Adaptation level theory*. New York: Harper & Row.

Kubler-Ross, E. (1969). *On death and drying*. New York: Macmillan.

Marriner-Tomey, A. (1994). *Nursing theorists and their work* (3rd ed.). St. Louis: Mosby.

Nungesser, L. G. (1978). *Homophobia and speech disruptions*. Unpublished manuscript.

Nungesser, L. G. (1979). *Homophobia prejudice in homosexual males*. Unpublished honors thesis, Stanford University, Palo Alto, CA.

Nungesser, L. G. (1983). *Homosexual acts, actors, and identities*. New York: Praeger.

Nuwayhid, K. A. (1991). Role transition, distance and conflict. In Sr. C. Roy & H. A. Andrews (Eds.), *The Roy adaptation model: The definitive statement* (pp. 363-376). Norwalk, CT: Appleton & Lange.

Phillips, K. D. (1994). *Testing biobehavioral adaptation in persons living with AIDS using Roy's theory of the person as an adaptive system.* Unpublished doctoral dissertation, The University of Tennessee, Knoxville, TN.

Rambo, B. (1984). *Adaptation nursing: Assessment and intervention.* Philadelphia: W. B. Saunders.

Randell, B., Poush Tedrow, M., & Van Landingham, J. (1982). *Adaptation nursing: The Roy conceptual model applied.* St. Louis: Mosby.

Roy, Sr. C. (1970). Adaptation: A conceptual framework for nursing. *Nursing Outlook, 18,* 43-45.

Roy, Sr. C. (1981). *Introduction to nursing: An adaptation model.* Englewood Cliffs, NJ: Prentice-Hall.

Roy, Sr. C., & Andrews, H. A. (1991). *The Roy adaptation model: The definitive statement.* Norwalk, CT: Appleton & Lange.

Task Force on Nutrition Support in AIDS (1989). Guidelines for nutrition support in AIDS. *Nutrition, 5*(1), 39-45.

Tedrow, M. P. (1991). Overview of the independence mode. In Sr. C. Roy & H. A. Andrews (Eds.), *The Roy adaptation model: The definitive statement* (pp. 385-403). Norwalk, CT: Appleton & Lange.

Welsh, M. D., & Clochesy, J. M. (Eds.). (1990). *Case studies in cardiovascular care nursing.* Rockville, MD: Aspen.

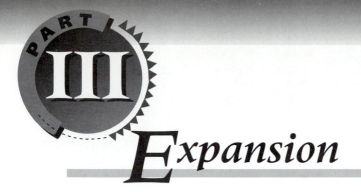

Expansion

Continued development of the substantive body of nursing knowledge is essential to the future of professional nursing practice.

- The utility of nursing models and theories of nursing as structures to guide critical nursing thought has been demonstrated.
- Areas of nursing practice for further theory application and development are plentiful.
- Nursing models and theories of nursing hold value for the discipline of nursing and professional nursing practice as we embrace the challenges of the new century.

Areas for Further Development of Theory-Based Nursing Practice

Martha Raile Alligood

"Systematic theory testing through application of nursing theories in practice with the participation of clinicians is essential for the enhancement of theory-based practice." *(Silva & Sorrell, 1992)*

Although practice based on nursing models and theories has been noted (see Chapter 2), there are many more areas of nursing practice that remain for theory development and expansion of theory-based practice. Bishop (1994) notes the plea of both scholars and practitioners for "increased attention to the relationships between theory and practice" (p. 56) and identifies these priorities:

1. Continued development of nursing theories that are relevant to the areas of practice engaged in by nurses
2. Increased use of nursing theories in clinical decision making
3. Increased collaboration between scientists and practitioners
4. Efforts by nurse researchers to communicate findings from research to relevant practitioners
5. Increased emphasis on clinical research

This text builds on Bishop's general concern: recognition of the importance of the relationship between theory and practice. The use of nursing models as critical thinking structures to guide clinical decision making (as presented in Chapters 1 and 3) addresses Bishop's second priority. This chapter focuses on her first priority and addresses it by (1) suggesting middle-range theories that can be derived from the grand theories of each model and (2) expanding the areas of nursing practice for their application.

New middle-range theories may be derived from models or grand theories that are relevant to specific areas of nursing practice. Middle-range theories are usually developed in relation to the specifics of actual clinical practice situations. However, ideas can be generated for new middle-range theory by using the grand theories to examine specific areas of nursing practice in which theory development is needed. Middle-range theory is more specific to practice (as discussed in Chapter 3), indicating the situation or health condition, client population or age group, location or area of practice, and action of the nurse or the intervention. These specifics make middle-range theory applicable to nursing practice.

The areas of nursing practice in which theory-based practice has been reported were presented in Tables 2-1, 2-2, and 2-3 in Chapter 2. In this chapter, these tables are reversed to indicate the areas in which theory-based practice has *not* been reported and to highlight opportunities for expansion. Table 11-1 presents areas for expansion in which practice with nursing models is described in terms of situation or health condition with a medical model focus. Table 11-2 presents areas for expansion in which practice with nursing models focuses on human development, type of practice, type of care, or health. Table 11-3 presents areas for expansion in which practice with nursing models focuses on a nursing intervention or nursing role.

JOHNSON

Middle-range theories may be derived from Johnson's behavioral system model and the grand theory of the person as a behavioral system. Tables 2-1, 2-2, and 2-3 in Chapter 2 reflect areas for expansion of Johnson's model in nursing practice. Since five applications of Johnson's model are included in the 49 situations or health conditions in Table 2-1, the 44 possible areas for expansion of Johnson's theory are listed in Table 11-1 (e.g., burns, leukemia, osteoporosis). Likewise, since five applications are included in the 32 areas in Table 2-2, there are 27 specific areas for expansion in Table 11-2, such as nursing of women, risk reduction, and rehabilitation. Table 2-3 includes practice with specific nursing interventions, and because none was reported with Johnson's model, there are 15 areas for expansion as noted in Table 11-3. Therefore, based on the information in Tables 11-1, 11-2, and 11-3, a middle-range theory from Johnson's grand theory might be the reduction of risk for osteoporosis through behavioral counseling.

TABLE 11-1 Areas of Practice for Expansion with Nursing Models Described in Terms of Medical Model Focus

Practice Areas	Johnson	King	Levine	Neuman	Orem	Rogers	Roy
Acute care	•	•	•	•	•		•
Adolescent cancer	•	•	•	•	•	•	
Adult diabetes	•		•	•		•	•
AIDS management		•	•		•		
Alzheimer's disease	•	•	•	•	•	•	
Ambulatory care	•	•	•	•			•
Anxiety	•		•	•		•	•
Breast cancer	•	•		•	•	•	
Burns	•	•		•		•	
Cancer	•	•		•			•
Cancer pain management		•	•	•	•	•	•
Cardiac disease	•		•	•		•	
Cardiomyopathy	•	•	•	•	•	•	
Chronic pain	•	•		•	•		•
Cognitive impairment	•	•	•		•	•	•
Congestive heart failure	•	•		•	•	•	•
Critical care	•	•					
Guillain-Barré syndrome	•	•	•	•		•	•
Heart variations	•	•	•	•	•		•
Hemodialysis		•	•	•		•	•
Hypernatremia	•	•	•	•	•		
Intensive care	•	•	•				
Kawasaki disease	•	•	•	•	•	•	
Leukemia	•	•	•	•	•	•	
Long-term care	•	•		•		•	•
Medical illness	•		•		•		•
Menopause	•		•	•	•		•
Neurofibromatosis	•		•	•	•	•	•
Oncology		•	•	•			•
Orthopedics	•		•		•	•	•
Osteoporosis	•	•	•	•	•	•	
Ostomy care	•	•	•	•		•	•
Pediatric	•	•	•	•	•		•
Perioperative	•	•		•	•	•	
Polio survivors	•	•	•	•	•		•
Postanesthesia	•	•	•	•	•	•	
Postpartum	•	•	•	•	•	•	
Posttrauma	•	•		•	•		
Preoperative adults	•	•		•	•		•
Preoperative anxiety	•		•	•		•	•
Pressure ulcers	•	•		•	•	•	•
Renal disease	•		•			•	•
Rheumatoid arthritis	•	•	•	•			
Schizophrenia	•	•	•	•	•	•	
Substance abuse	•	•	•	•			•
Terminal illness	•	•	•	•	•		
Ventilator patient	•	•	•	•	•		
Ventricular tachycardia		•	•	•	•	•	•
Wound healing	•	•		•	•	•	•

TABLE 11-2   Areas for Expansion with Nursing Models Based on Human Development, Type of Practice, Type of Care, or Type of Health

Practice Areas	Johnson	King	Levine	Neuman	Orem	Rogers	Roy
Cesarean father	•	•	•	•	•	•	
Child health	•		•	•	•	•	•
Child psychiatric	•	•	•		•	•	•
Dying process	•	•	•	•			•
Emergency	•				•	•	
Gerontology	•		•				
High-risk infants	•		•	•	•	•	•
Holistic care	•	•		•	•	•	•
Homeless	•	•		•	•	•	•
Hospice	•	•		•		•	•
Managed care	•		•	•	•	•	•
Mental health		•	•				•
Neonates	•	•	•	•	•	•	
Nursing administration	•		•				•
Nursing adolescents			•	•		•	•
Nursing adults	•						•
Nursing children		•		•			
Nursing community			•				
Nursing elderly	•						
Nursing families	•		•		•		•
Nursing home residents	•	•	•	•	•	•	
Nursing infants	•	•		•		•	
Nursing in space	•	•	•	•			•
Nursing service	•	•	•	•	•		•
Nursing women	•	•	•	•			•
Occupational health	•	•	•	•		•	•
Palliative care	•	•	•	•	•	•	•
Psychiatric nursing	•	•	•	•	•		•
Public health	•	•	•		•	•	•
Quality assurance		•	•	•	•	•	•
Rehabilitation	•	•					
Risk reduction	•	•			•	•	•

KING

Middle-range theories may be derived from King's theory of goal attainment. The details of the actual clinical situation specify the theory; however, use of Tables 11-1, 11-2, and 11-3 may help identify areas for expansion of King's theory for nursing practice. Nine of the 49 areas listed in Table 2-1 reported the use of King's theory, so there are 40 health conditions for possible expansion in Table 11-1, such as breast

TABLE 11-3	Areas for Expansion of Nursing Intervention or Role						
Practice Areas	**Johnson**	**King**	**Levine**	**Neuman**	**Orem**	**Rogers**	**Roy**
Breastfeeding	•	•	•		•	•	
Community presence	•	•	•	•	•		•
Counseling	•	•	•	•	•		•
Family therapy	•		•		•	•	•
Group therapy	•		•	•	•		
Health patterning	•	•	•	•	•		•
Imagery	•	•	•	•	•		•
Intentionality	•	•	•	•	•		•
Knowing participation	•	•	•	•	•		•
Life-patterning difficulties	•	•	•	•	•		•
Life review	•	•	•	•	•		•
Nutrition	•	•	•		•	•	•
Parenting	•		•		•	•	
Storytelling	•	•	•	•	•		•
Therapeutic touch	•	•	•	•	•		•

cancer, postpartum, and substance abuse. In Table 2-2, 11 of the 32 client groups or areas of practice were represented by publications based on King's theory, which leaves 21 areas of practice for expansion in Table 11-2, such as hospice, occupational health, and nursing of women. Three of the 15 nursing interventions in Table 2-3 were King theory–based interventions, leaving 12 areas for possible expansion in Table 11-3 (e.g., health patterning, life review, parenting). Therefore a middle-range theory from King's theory of goal attainment might be mutual goal setting and health patterning in postpartum women leads to goal attainment.

LEVINE

Middle-range theories may be derived from Levine's theory of therapeutic intention. The details of actual clinical situations specify the theory; however, Tables 11-1, 11-2, and 11-3 may be used to stimulate thinking and expand the use of Levine's model in practice. Ten of the 49 were applications of Levine's model in Table 2-1, leaving 39 areas for expansion in Table 11-1 (e.g., hemodialysis, posttrauma, ostomy care). Nine of the 32 client groups or areas of practice reported using Levine's model in Table 2-2, leaving 23 areas for expansion as noted in Table 11-2, such as nursing of adolescents, gerontology, and homeless. Specific nursing interventions were not found based on Levine's model in Table 2-3, so Table 11-3 lists 15 areas for possible expansion. A middle-range theory derived from Levine's theory of therapeutic intention might be therapeutic regimens that facilitate holistic adaptation of adolescents in posttrauma foster their health.

NEUMAN

Middle-range theories may be derived from Neuman's theory of optimal client stability. The details of actual clinical situations specify the theory; however, Tables 11-1, 11-2, and 11-3 lead to ideas for possible expansion. Seven of the 49 conditions were reported in nursing practice guided by the Neuman model in Table 2-1, so there are 42 areas of practice in Table 11-1 for expansion, such as Alzheimer's, rheumatoid arthritis, and hemodialysis. Twelve of the 32 client groups or areas of practice in Table 2-2 were addressed in publications based on Neuman's model, leaving 20 areas for expansion as noted in Table 11-2 (e.g., occupational health, psychiatric nursing, quality assurance). Four of 15 nursing interventions were reported in Table 2-3 using the Neuman model; therefore there are 11 areas for possible expansion listed in Table 11-3, such as group therapy, storytelling, and life-patterning difficulties. A middle-range theory derived from Neuman's theory of optimal client stability might be occupational health of rheumatoid arthritis patients is stabilized by identifying stressors that lead to life-patterning difficulties.

OREM

Middle-range theories are derived from Orem's self-care deficit or dependent-care theory. The details of actual clinical situations provide the specifics of the theory; however, Tables 11-1, 11-2, and 11-3 may be used to stimulate thinking for theory expansion. Use of Orem's model in practice was reported in 17 of the 49 areas included in Table 2-1, leaving 32 areas for possible expansion in Table 11-1, such as AIDS management, breast cancer, and leukemia. Although 13 of the 32 client groups or areas of practice were addressed in publications based on Orem's theory in Table 2-2, 19 areas for expansion remain in Table 11-2 (e.g., child health, nursing of families, the dying process). Specific interventions based on Orem as reported in Table 2-3 were not found, therefore the 15 areas of possible expansion are noted in Table 11-3. A middle-range theory derived from Orem's self-care deficit theory might specify preserving self-care in AIDS patients in the dying process through nutrition.

ROGERS

Middle-range theories may be derived from Rogers' theory of accelerating change. The details from actual clinical situations specify the theory; however, ideas for theory expansion are generated from Tables 11-1, 11-2, and 11-3. Fifteen of the 49 conditions included in Table 2-1 were addressed by nurses whose practice was guided by Rogerian science, leaving 34 areas for possible expansion listed in Table 11-1 (e.g., adolescent cancer, orthopedics, chronic pain). Nurses reported practice in 15 of the 32 client groups or areas of practice in Table 2-2, which means there are 17 areas for possible expansion listed in Table 11-2, such as nursing adolescents, nursing infants, and palliative care. Eleven of the 15 interventions in Table 2-3 were based on nursing practice with Rogers; therefore there are four areas for expansion in Table 11-3, such as breastfeeding, parenting, and group therapy. A middle-range theory derived from Rogers' theory of accelerating change might be patients with chronic pain identify group therapy as a measure that is palliative to its onset.

ROY

Middle-range theories may be derived from Roy's theory of the person as an adaptive system. The details from actual clinical practice normally generate the specifics of the theory; however, ideas for theory expansion are developed in Tables 11-1, 11-2, and 11-3 that reflect new areas for theory-based practice. Nineteen of the 49 health conditions were addressed by nurses practicing with Roy's model in Table 2-1, leaving 30 areas for expansion listed in Table 11-1, such as anxiety, cardiac disease, and oncology. Ten of the 32 client groups or areas of practice in Table 2-2 were included in publications based on Roy's model, which means there are 22 areas for expansion in Table 11-2, such as nursing adolescents, holistic care, and nursing of women. Two of the 15 nursing interventions in Table 2-3 were based on Roy's model, leaving 13 areas for expansion in Table 11-3 (e.g., imagery, nutrition, intentionality). A middle-range theory derived from Roy's theory of the person as an adaptive system might be adolescents experiencing anxiety adapt through the intervention of imagery and improve their coping.

CONCLUSION

This chapter addresses Bishop's first priority by suggesting additional middle-range theories and possible new areas for theory-based practice. As noted in Chapter 1, nursing has gone through numerous eras with different nursing knowledge emphases. This text acknowledges the shift from theory development to theory utilization in this theory era. The shift ushers in a challenge to nurses to move beyond the focus of the nursing process and nursing action to one of application of theories relative to the *patient* in theory-based practice. The nursing models and theories have been set forth and demonstrated to be decision-making structures that guide nursing practice (in Chapters 4 to 10). Smith (1993) has pointed out that "some knowledge base or perspective guides all nursing practice" (p. 8). The importance of further development of theory-based nursing practice to the development of the discipline cannot be overemphasized.

References

Bishop, S. (1994). Theory development process. In A. Marriner-Tomey, (Ed.), *Nursing theorists and their work* (pp. 45-57). St. Louis: Mosby.

Silva, M., & Sorrell, J. (1992). Testing of nursing theory: Critique and philosophical expansion. *Advances in Nursing Science, 14*(4), 12-23.

Smith, M. (1993). Case management and nursing theory-based practice. *Nursing Science Quarterly, 6*(1), 8-9.

Conceptual Models of Nursing, Nursing Theories, and Nursing Practice: Focus on the Future

Jacqueline Fawcett

"The discipline of nursing can survive and advance only if nurses celebrate their own heritage and acknowledge their own knowledge base by adopting explicit conceptual models of nursing and nursing theories to guide their activities." (Fawcett, 1995)

Nursing knowledge, in the form of conceptual models of nursing and nursing theories, has been developed by several nurse scholars who have devoted a great deal of time to observing clinical situations, thinking about what is important to *nursing* in those situations, and then publishing their ideas in books, book chapters, and journal articles. Nursing knowledge continues to evolve as nursing students, clinicians, and researchers use those conceptual models and theories to guide their clinical practice and research and then report the results at conferences and in publications. Thus all nurses can contribute to the evolution of nursing knowledge and the subsequent advancement of nursing practice.

The purpose of this chapter is to focus on the future of conceptual models of nursing and nursing theories for nursing practice. The chapter begins with a discussion of the philosophic value of using explicit nursing models and theories to guide nursing practice. Next, strategies that can be adopted by the individual nurse to implement nursing model–based and nursing theory–based nursing practice are identified. Recommendations for the work that is needed to determine the scientific value of conceptual models of nursing and nursing theories are then offered.

PHILOSOPHIC VALUE OF USING EXPLICIT NURSING KNOWLEDGE

The future influence of nursing knowledge on nursing practice is promising. The current recognition of the value of using explicit nursing models and theories to guide nursing practice is documented in numerous publications, many of which are listed at the end of Chapter 2 of this book. At the same time, however, the rapid growth of nurse practitioner programs has diverted attention away from nursing knowledge and toward medical knowledge as the base for practice. The result is that some nurses have rejected the knowledge of their own discipline as they strive to become "junior doctors" instead of "senior nurses" (Meleis, 1993). Consequently, the value of using nursing knowledge to guide nursing practice needs to be underscored.

Every nurse uses knowledge gained from formal study and practical experience to guide practice. The knowledge used, however, tends to be implicit. That is, the nurse typically is not aware of what knowledge is being used or its source. Unfortunately, implicit knowledge tends to be "disconnected, diffused, incomplete and frequently heavily weighted by concepts drawn from the conceptual schema used by medicine to achieve its own social mission" (Johnson, 1987, p. 195).

The explicit use of conceptual models of nursing and nursing theories to guide nursing practice is the hallmark of professional nursing. The use of *nursing* models and theories "distinguishes nursing as an autonomous health profession" and represents "nursing's unique contribution to the health care system" (Parse, 1995, p. 128). Furthermore, Anderson (1995) pointed out that the use of a "well-developed body of knowledge distinguishes a profession from a trade" (p. 247). She went on to explain that as a professional discipline, nursing "must ensure that we have a solid scholarly and scientific foundation upon which to base our practice" (p. 247). It is therefore incumbent on all nurses to use explicit conceptual models of nursing and nursing theories and to evaluate that use in a systematic manner.

Research findings indicate that nurses feel vulnerable and experience a great deal of stress as they attempt to achieve professional aspirations within a rapidly changing, medically dominated, and bureaucratic healthcare delivery system (Graham, 1994). As structures for critical thinking within a *distinctively nursing* context, conceptual models of nursing and nursing theories provide the intellectual skills that nurses need to survive at a time when cost containment through reduction of professional nursing staff is the modus operandi of the administrators of healthcare delivery systems.

Feeg (1989) and Fawcett (1995) have explained that the conceptual models of nursing and nursing theories collectively identify the distinctive nursing territory within the vast arena of healthcare. Each nursing model and theory provides a holistic orientation that reminds nurses of the focus of the discipline—concern for the "wholeness or health of humans, recognizing that humans are in continuous interaction with their environments" (Donaldson & Crowley, 1978, p. 119). Furthermore, each conceptual model of nursing and nursing theory provides a *nursing* lens for viewing clinical situations and facilitates the identification of details that are relevant to nursing from the plethora of available information. In addition, nursing models and theories help nurses to explicate what they know and why they do what they do. In other words, nursing models and theories facilitate the communication of nursing knowledge and how that knowledge governs the actions performed on behalf of or in conjunction with people who require healthcare. Ultimately, then, nursing practice that is based on an explicit conceptual model or nursing theory is "for our patients' sake" (Dabbs, 1994, p. 220).

IMPLEMENTING NURSING KNOWLEDGE–BASED NURSING PRACTICE: PROCESS AND STRATEGIES

The substantive and process elements of implementing conceptual model–based nursing practice at the clinical agency level have been discussed in detail by Fawcett (1995). In this chapter, the focus narrows to the process that occurs and the strategies that can be used by the individual nurse when implementing a conceptual model of nursing–based or nursing theory–based nursing practice. Understanding and telling others about the process and using the strategies now should ensure that *nursing* knowledge is used to guide practice in the future.

In Chapters 1 and 3 of this book, Alligood points out that the first step toward conceptual model of nursing–based or nursing theory–based nursing practice is "the decision to do so." That decision certainly was made by the authors of Chapters 4 through 10 of this book.

The second step is to recognize that the adoption of an explicit conceptual model of nursing or nursing theory—or a change from one explicit model or theory to another—requires an adjustment in thinking about clinical situations. More specifically, the successful implementation of the conceptual model of nursing–based or nursing theory–based nursing practice requires recognition of the fact that the nurse needs time to evolve from the use of one frame of reference for practice to another frame of reference. Time is required regardless of whether the original frame of reference is an implicit one or a different explicit model or theory. The process that occurs during the period of evolution is referred to as *perspective transformation*.

Perspective Transformation

Drawing from Mezirow's early work in the development of adult learning theory (1975, 1978), Rogers (1989) (a Canadian nurse who is not related to the author of the science of unitary human beings) explained that perspective transformation is based on the assumption that "individuals have a personal paradigm or meaning perspective that structures the way in which they existentially experience, interpret, and understand their world" (p. 112). She defined and described perspective transformation as the process

> whereby the assumptions, values, and beliefs that constitute a given meaning perspective come to consciousness, are reflected upon, and are critically analyzed. The process involves gradually taking on a new perspective along with the corresponding assumptions, values, and beliefs. The new perspective gives rise to fundamental structural changes in the way individuals see themselves and their relationships with others, leading to a reinterpretation of their personal, social, or occupational worlds. (Rogers, 1989, p. 112)

Thus the process of perspective transformation involves the shift from one meaning perspective or frame of reference about nursing and nursing practice to another, from one way "of viewing and being with human beings" to another (Nagle & Mitchell, 1991, p. 22).

Rogers pointed out that the cognitive and emotional aspects of perspective transformation represent "dramatic individual change for every nurse" (1989, p. 112). Moreover, she underscored the importance of recognizing, appreciating, and acknowledging that during the process of perspective transformation, each nurse evolves from feeling "a [profound] sense of loss followed by an ultimate sense of liberation and empowerment" (1992, p. 23). Clearly, perspective transformation requires considerable effort and a strong commitment to change (Nagle & Mitchell, 1991).

Perspective transformation encompasses nine phases: stability, dissonance, confusion, dwelling with uncertainty, saturation, synthesis, resolution, reconceptualization, and return to stability (Rogers, 1992). The prevailing period of *stability* is disrupted when the idea of implementing conceptual model–based or nursing theory–based nursing practice or changing the model or theory is introduced. *Dissonance* occurs as the nurse begins to examine his/her current frame of reference for practice in light of the challenge to adopt or change a conceptual model or theory. As the nurse begins to learn the content of the new conceptual model or theory, the discrepancies between the current way of practice and what nursing practice could be begins to be appreciated. A phase of *confusion* follows. As the nurse struggles to learn more about the model or theory and its implications for practice, a feeling of "lying in limbo" between frames of reference prevails (Rogers, 1992, p. 22). Throughout the phases of dissonance and confusion, the nurse frequently feels anxious, angry, and unable to think. Rogers (1992) explained that these distressing emotions "seem to arise out of the grieving of a loss of an intimate part of the self. The existing [frame of reference] no longer makes sense, yet the new [model or theory] is not sufficiently internalized to provide resolution" (p. 22).

The phase of confusion is followed by the phase of *dwelling with uncertainty*. At this point, the nurse acknowledges that confusion "is not a result of some personal inadequacy" (Rogers, 1992, p. 22). As a consequence, anxiety is replaced by a "feeling of freedom to critically examine old ways and explore the new [model or theory]" (Rogers, 1992, p. 22). The phase of dwelling with uncertainty is spent immersed in information that frequently seems obscure and irrelevant. It is a time of "wallowing in the obscure while waiting for moments of coherence that lead to unity of thought" (Smith, 1988, p. 3).

The phase of *saturation* occurs when the nurse feels that he/she "cannot think about or learn anything more about the nursing [model or theory]" (Rogers, 1992, p. 22). The phase does not represent resistance but rather "the need to separate from the difficult process of transformation, [which] is part of the natural ebb and flow of the learning experience" (Rogers, 1992, p. 22).

The phase of *synthesis* occurs as insights render the content of the new conceptual model or theory coherent and meaningful. The formerly obscure practice implications of the conceptual model or theory become clear and worthy of the implementation effort. Increasing tension is followed by exhilaration as insights illuminate the connections between the content of the conceptual model or theory and its use in nursing practice (Rogers, 1992; Smith, 1988). "These insights," Smith (1988) explained, "are moments of coherence, flashes of unity, as though suddenly the fog lifts and clarity prevails. These moments of coherence push one beyond to deepened levels of understanding" (p. 3).

The phase of *resolution* is characterized by "a feeling of comfort with the new nursing [model or theory]. The feelings of dissonance and discontent . . . are resolved and the anxiety is dissipated" (Rogers, 1992, p. 23). During this phase, "nurses describe themselves as changed, as seeing the world differently and feeling a distinct sense of empowerment" (Rogers, 1992, p. 23).

The phase of *reconceptualization* occurs as the nurse consciously reconceptualizes nursing practice using the new conceptual model of nursing or nursing theory (Rogers, 1992). During this phase, the nurse compares the activities of practice, from patient assessment through shift reports, according to the old and new ways of thinking and changes those activities so that they are in keeping with the new model or theory. The final phase, *return to stability,* occurs when nursing practice is clearly based on the new conceptual model of nursing or nursing theory.

Strategies to Facilitate Perspective Transformation

Rogers (1989) identified several strategies that can be used to facilitate perspective transformation. These strategies are especially effective during the early phases of perspective transformation when the nurse is experiencing a move from the original to the new frame of reference for practice.

One strategy is to use analogies to facilitate understanding of the terms, conceptual model, and theory. Such analogies as chair or book can be used for concepts (conceptual), the analogy of a model home or model airplane can be used for model, and the analogy of a conjecture can be used for theory. Rogers (1989) noted that the acts of conceptualizing and theorizing can be demystified "by stating that it is not a process reserved for intellectuals, but rather a cognitive process of all humans that begins in infancy as a baby puts together all the pieces to form the concept of mother" (p. 114).

Two other strategies are directed toward identification of the nurse's existing frame of reference for nursing practice. One of those strategies is to list words that reflect the nurse's view of nursing practice. Similarly, the nurse could depict his/her view of nursing practice in drawings or collages of photographs. Another strategy is to think about the details of, reasons for, and outcomes of a recent interaction with a patient.

Once the nurse has gained a clear understanding of the original frame of reference, he/she needs to explore the difference between the current state of nursing practice and what practice would be like using the new conceptual model or theory. This can be accomplished through the use of provocative strategies. One provocative strategy is to think about how such situations as childbirth and death are currently managed and how they could be managed using the new model or theory. Another strategy is to describe what is unique about nursing practice or what would be done if physicians' orders did not have to be followed.

Rogers (1989) pointed out that as the nurse becomes aware of the differences between the present and the potential future practice of nursing, he/she experiences a cognitive dissonance or discomfort that comes from "the awareness of the 'what is' versus 'what [c]ould be'" (p. 115). She concluded by noting that when cognitive dissonance "has been experienced by nurses both individually or collectively, then perspective transformation can occur and a climate for the implementation of a nursing [model or theory] will have been created" (p. 116).

Subsequent stages of perspective transformation and the implementation of conceptual model–based or theory–based nursing practice are facilitated by constant reinforcement. Accordingly, all nursing activities should be tied to the conceptual model or theory in a systematic manner. The novice user of an explicit conceptual model or theory should not become discouraged if initial experiences seem forced or awkward. Adoption of an explicit conceptual model of nursing or nursing theory does require restructuring the nurse's way of thinking about clinical situations and use of a new vocabulary. However, repeated use of the model or theory should lead to more systematic and organized endeavors. Regarding this, Broncatello (1980, p. 23) commented,

> The nurse's consistent use of any model [or theory] for the interpretation of observable client data is most definitely not an easy task. Much like the development of any habitual behavior, it initially requires thought, discipline and the gradual evolvement of a mind set of what is important to observe within the guidelines of the model [or theory]. As is true of most habits, however, it makes decision making less complicated.

SCIENTIFIC VALUE OF USING EXPLICIT NURSING KNOWLEDGE

The scientific value of using conceptual models of nursing and nursing theories as guides for nursing practice has begun to be documented in the form of the credibility of each conceptual model and the empirical adequacy of each theory. Inasmuch as a review of the relevant literature is beyond the scope of this chapter, readers are referred to extensive evaluations in *Analysis and Evaluation of Nursing Theories* (Fawcett, 1993), and *Analysis and Evaluation of Conceptual Models of Nursing* (Fawcett, 1995). Much more work is needed, however.

Documentation of Nursing Practice

The methodology of nursing practice is operationalized by the documents and technology used to guide and direct nursing practice, to record observations and results of interventions, and to describe and evaluate nursing job performance. In other words, the methodology encompasses the standards for nursing care, department and unit objectives, nursing care plans, patient database and classification tools, flow sheets, Kardex forms, computer information systems, quality assurance tools, nursing job description and performance appraisal tools, and other relevant documents and technologies (Fawcett, 1992; Fitch et al., 1991; Laurie-Shaw & Ives, 1988; Weiss & Teplick, 1993/1995). Each existing document and all current technology must be reviewed for its congruence with the conceptual model of nursing or nursing theory and revised as necessary. Although revisions frequently are needed and the work may seem overwhelming at the outset, the importance of having documents and technologies that are congruent with the conceptual model or theory cannot be overemphasized. In fact, this congruence may be regarded as the sine qua non of conceptual model–based or theory-based nursing practice. Although at least one computer software program (Bliss-Holtz, Taylor, & McLaughlin, 1992) and many documentation tools (Fawcett, 1993, 1995; Weiss & Teplick, 1993/1995) have been developed, systematic studies are needed to determine the utility of the software and the validity and reliability of the tools.

Communicating the Scope and Substance of Nursing Practice

The decision to implement conceptual model–based or theory-based nursing practice typically is undertaken in response to the quest for a way to articulate the substance and scope of professional nursing practice to other healthcare disciplines and the public and to improve the conditions and outcomes of nursing practice. Consequently, one potential outcome of conceptual model–based or theory-based nursing practice is enhanced understanding of the role of nursing in healthcare by administrators, physicians, social workers, dietitians, physical therapists, occupational therapists, respiratory therapists, and other healthcare team members, as well as by recipients of nursing. Research is needed to determine the extent to which the role of nursing within the healthcare delivery system is better understood when practice is based on an explicit conceptual model of nursing or nursing theory.

Measuring Satisfaction

Another potential outcome is the nurse's increased satisfaction with the conditions and outcomes of his/her nursing practice through an explicit focus on and identification of *nursing* problems and actions, as well as through enhanced communication and documentation (Fitch et al., 1991). Still another potential outcome is increased satisfaction of patients and their families with the nursing that is received. The evidence regarding nurse, patient, and family satisfaction is primarily in the form of anecdotal reports from just a few clinical agencies (e.g., Scherer, 1988; Studio Three, 1992). A plethora of instruments have been designed to measure nurse and patient satisfaction. Only a few of these instruments, however, measure satisfaction with nursing practice that is based on an explicit conceptual model of nursing or nursing theory (e.g., Marckx, 1995). Thus valid and reliable instruments need to be developed before systematic, multisite studies, which are necessary to document nurse, patient, and family satisfaction, are undertaken.

Utility of Nursing Models and Theories Across Populations

The literature associated with the seven conceptual models included in this book suggests that each model is appropriate in a wide range of nursing specialties and for many different populations of nursing recipients (see Chapters 2 and 11). Aggleton and Chalmers (1985) noted that the literature "might encourage some nurses to feel that it does not really matter which model of nursing is chosen to inform nursing practice within a particular care setting" (p. 39). They also noted that that literature might "encourage the view that choosing between models is something one does intuitively, as an act of personal preference. Even worse, it might encourage some nurses to feel that all their everyday problems might be eliminated were they to make the 'right choice' in selecting a particular model for use across a care setting" (p. 39).

Critical appraisals of the literature have not yet revealed the extent to which the fit of the conceptual model or theory to particular populations of nursing recipients might have been forced. In fact, the issue of forced fit has not yet been addressed in the literature. Clearly, this is necessary future research.

Furthermore, little attention has been given to the extent to which a particular conceptual model or theory is modified to fit a given situation (C.P. Germain, personal communication, October 21, 1987). Although modifications certainly are acceptable, they should be acknowledged, and serious consideration should be given to renaming the conceptual model or theory to indicate that modifications have been made. Clearly, systematic exploration of the nursing clinical specialty practice implications of various conceptual models, coupled with more practical experience with each model and theory in a variety of settings, is required.

CONCLUSION

The belief that explicit conceptual models of nursing and nursing theories, rather than medical models and theories, are the proper guides for nursing practice has permeated the discussion. The continued use of medical knowledge, coupled with a rejection of nursing knowledge, reflects the thinking of an oppressed group (Bent, 1993). Nurses must therefore break the intellectual chains associated with self-imposed oppression by rejecting medical knowledge as the fundamental basis of nursing practice.

References

Aggleton, P., & Chalmers, H. (1985). Critical examination. *Nursing Times, 81*(14), 38-39.

Anderson, C. A. (1995). Scholarship: How important is it? [Editorial]. *Nursing Outlook, 43,* 247-248.

Bent, K. N. (1993). Perspectives on critical and feminist theory in developing nursing praxis. *Journal of Professional Nursing, 9,* 296-303.

Bliss-Holtz, J., Taylor, S. G., & McLaughlin, K. (1992). Nursing theory as a base for computerized nursing information system. *Nursing Science Quarterly, 5,* 124-128.

Broncatello, K. F. (1980). Auger in action: Application of the model. *Advances in Nursing Science, 2*(2), 13-23.

Dabbs, A. D. V. (1994). Theory-based nursing practice: For our patients' sake. *Clinical Nurse Specialist, 8,* 214, 220.

Donaldson, S. K., & Crowley, D. M. (1978). The discipline of nursing. *Nursing Outlook, 26,* 113-120.

Fawcett, J. (1992). Conceptual models and nursing practice: The reciprocal relationship. *Journal of Advanced Nursing, 17,* 224-228.

Fawcett, J. (1993). *Analysis and evaluation of nursing theories.* Philadelphia: F. A. Davis.

Fawcett, J. (1995). *Analysis and evaluation of conceptual models of nursing* (3rd ed.). Philadelphia: F. A. Davis.

Feeg, V. (1989). Is theory application merely an intellectual exercise? [Editorial]. *Pediatric Nursing, 15,* 450.

Fitch, M., Rogers, M., Ross, E., Shea, H., Smith, I., & Tucker, D. (1991). Developing a plan to evaluate the use of nursing conceptual frameworks. *Canadian Journal of Nursing Administration, 4*(1), 22-28.

Graham, I. (1994). How do registered nurses think and experience nursing: A phenomenological investigation. *Journal of Clinical Nursing, 3,* 235-242.

Johnson, D. E. (1987). Evaluating conceptual models for use in critical care nursing practice. [Guest editorial]. *Dimensions of Critical Care Nursing, 6,* 195-197.

Laurie-Shaw, B., & Ives, S. M. (1988). Implementing Orem's self-care deficit theory: Part II—Adopting a conceptual framework of nursing. *Canadian Journal of Nursing Administration, 1*(2), 16-19.

Marckx, B. B. (1995). Watson's theory of caring: A model for implementation in practice. *Journal of Nursing Care Quality, 9*(4), 43-54.

Meleis, A. I. (1993, April). *Nursing research and the Neuman model: Directions for the future.* Panel discussion with B. Neuman, A. I. Meleis, J. Fawcett, L. Lowry, M. C. Smith, & A. Edgil conducted at the Fourth Biennial International Neuman Systems Model Symposium, Rochester, NY.

Mezirow, J. (1975). *Education for perspective transformation: Women's re-entry programs in community colleges.* New York: Center for Adult Education, Teachers College, Columbia University.

Mezirow, J. (1978). Perspective transformation. *Adult Education, 28,* 100-110.

Nagle, L. M., & Mitchell, G. J. (1991). Theoretic diversity: Evolving paradigmatic issues in research and practice. *Advances in Nursing Science, 14*(1), 17-25.

Parse, R. R. (1995). Commentary. Parse's theory of human becoming: An alternative guide to nursing practice for pediatric oncology nurses. *Journal of Pediatric Oncology Nursing, 12,* 128.

Rogers, M. E. (1989). Creating a climate for the implementation of a nursing conceptual framework. *Journal of Continuing Education in Nursing, 20,* 112-116.

Rogers, M. E. (1992, February-April). *Transformative learning: Understanding and facilitating nurses' learning of nursing conceptual frameworks.* Paper presented at Sigma Theta Tau Conferences, "Improving Practice and Education Through Theory." Chicago, IL; Pittsburgh, PA; Wilkes-Barre, PA.

Scherer, P. (1988). Hospitals that attract (and keep) nurses. *American Journal of Nursing, 88,* 34-40.

Smith, M. J. (1988). Wallowing while waiting. *Nursing Science Quarterly, 1,* 3.

Studio Three. (1992). *The nurse theorists: Excellence in action—Callista Roy.* Fuld Institute of Technology in Nursing Education, Athens, OH.

Weiss, M. E., & Teplick, F. (1993). Linking perinatal standards, documentation, and quality monitoring. *Journal of Perinatal and Neonatal Nursing, 7*(2), 18-27. [Reprinted in *Neonatal Intensive Care, 8*(1), 38-43, 58, 1995.]

Glossary

adaptation Process of change whereby individuals retain their integrity, or wholeness, with the realities of their environment. It is an expression of the integration of the entire organism.

agency Ability, capability, or power to engage in action in Orem's conceptual model.

basic conditioning factors (BCFs) Factors identified by Orem that influence individual health-related demands and the ability to engage in self-care (e.g., age, gender, health state, and family patterns).

behavioral system balance State in which a system is able to maintain a certain level of behavior within an acceptable range; stability; steady state.

behavioral system imbalance State in which there are disturbances in structure, function, or functional requirements in one or more subsystem that may be described in terms of insufficiency, discrepancy, dominance, or incompatibility.

central (centrality) Focal, pivotal, principal, or essential.

change Essence of life or process of adaptation that is directed, purposeful, meaningful, and imminently understandable.

conceptual models Group of related concepts that provides a broad frame of reference for systematic approaches to the phenomena with which the discipline is concerned; also known as frameworks or paradigms.

conceptualization Process of creative thinking that involves imagination, invention, contemplation, consideration, reflection, judgment, and conclusion.

conservation Keeping-together function of the nurse specified by Levine as a product of adaptation.

criteria for a profession Set of standards that a discipline or group uses as a gauge to recognize its level of development.

criterion   Standard by which something is measured or evaluated.

critical thinking   Disciplined process in which one actively and skillfully uses reason and logic in decision making as a guide to belief and action.

critical thinking structures   Conceptual or theoretical frameworks that guide the reasoning process and lead to decisive action.

developmental self-care requisites   Needs or goals that arise from maturational changes in the life cycle, such as pregnancy, or from situational events throughout human development, such as the death of a significant other.

deduction   Approach to thinking and reasoning that proceeds from the general to the particular.

diagnostic statement   Product of the assessment process in Neuman's systems model that reflects systematic consideration of actual or potential environmental stressors.

disequilibrium   Absence of client system balance in Neuman's systems model.

external regulatory force   Role of the nurse specified by Johnson to preserve the organization and integration of the client's behavior at an optimal level under conditions when the client's behavior constitutes a threat to physical and psychosocial health.

functional requirements/sustenal imperatives   Protection, nurturance, and stimulation that the behavioral system must receive from the environment to survive and develop.

grand theory   Proposition derived from a conceptual model or framework that is at a sufficiently high level of abstraction to enable the development of many middle-range applications that are specific to practice level details.

health deviation self-care requisites   Self-care deficits that arise when persons are ill or injured, have defects or disabilities, or are undergoing diagnosis or treatment.

induction   Approach to thinking and reasoning that proceeds from the particular to the general.

manifestation   What is perceivable of field patterning (Rogers) or the aspect of the field that one's perceptions can recognize.

metaparadigm   Global concepts that identify the phenomena of interest for a discipline.

middle-range theory   Least abstract set of related concepts that proposes a truth specific to the details of nursing practice.

mutual patterning   Process by which the human/environmental field process evolves; known patterns are identified in the human/environmental field process.

nursing art   Expressive and skillful activities of nursing tailored by the nurse's actions, blending knowledge with personal preferences.

nursing science   Knowledge of practice produced through the unique interrelationship of theory and research in approaches aimed at understanding the phenomena of interest to the discipline.

perceived dissonance Perception of disharmony or discomfort in the human/environmental field process in Rogers' model.

perspective transformation Process whereby the assumptions, values, and beliefs that constitute a given meaning perspective come to consciousness, are reflected on, and are critically analyzed. The process involves gradually taking on a new perspective along with the corresponding fundamental structural changes in the way individuals see themselves and their relationships with others, leading to a reinterpretation of personal, social, or occupational worlds. The nine phases of perspective transformation are stability, dissonance, confusion, dwelling with uncertainty, saturation, synthesis, resolution, reconceptualization, and return to stability.

provocative facts Presenting symptoms alerting one to a problem.

scholarship Development and communication of knowledge.

self-care deficit When self-care ability of a person is not adequate to meet the therapeutic self-care demand.

spiritual distress Disruption of the human spirit. The human spirit is that which gives meaning and purpose to life, serves to integrate the whole human being, and connects the individual to self, others, the universe, and the Creator. In spiritual distress, the individual may lose sight of the meaning and purpose of life or connectedness.

stability Equilibrium or client system balance in Neuman's systems model.

stressor Intrapersonal, interpersonal, or extrapersonal condition or situation identified by Neuman as a threat to the stability or integrity of the client system.

substantive Substantial, essential, having a solid basis, or independent in existence.

subsystem Minisystem with its own unique goal and function that is maintained as long as its relationship to other subsystems is in a steady state, functional requirements are provided, and the environment is not disturbed.

theory Group of related concepts that proposes actions that guide practice.

theory application Operation of a system of ideas in action.

theory development Knowledge-building process in the context of syntax, structure, and growth.

theory utilization Orchestration of a system of ideas for a purpose.

trophicognosis Nursing care judgment arrived at through the use of the scientific process (Levine).

universal self-care requisites Human needs for self-care that promote structural and functional integrity of the person and well-being, including maintenance of air, food, water, and elimination; balance between activity and rest; solitude and social interaction; prevention of hazards; and promotion of normalcy.

Index

A

Accelerating change, theory of, 38
Achievement assessment in Johnson's behavioral system model, 59
Acquired immunodeficiency syndrome (AIDS), 39, 190-198
Action in Johnson's behavioral system model, 51
Adaptation in Levine's conservation model, 90-91
Adaptation model, Roy's; *see* Roy's adaptation model
Adaptive system, person as, theory of, 39
Affiliative assessment in Johnson's behavioral system model, 60
Aggressive/protective assessment in Johnson's behavioral system model, 60
Aging, theory of, 38
AIDS; *see* Acquired immunodeficiency syndrome
American Journal of Nursing (AJN), 4
American Nurses Association (ANA), 6, 17
Analysis
  in King's systems framework and theory, 77
  and synthesis of data; *see* Synthesis and analysis of data
Application, 47-200
  Johnson's behavioral system model and, 49-70
  King's systems framework and, 71-88
  Levine's conservation model and, 89-107
  Neuman's systems model and, 109-127
  Orem's self-care deficit theory and, 129-152

Application—cont'd
  Rogers' science of unitary human beings and, 153-174
  Roy's adaptation model and, 175-200
Assessment
  behavioral; *see* Behavioral assessment
  in Johnson's behavioral system model, 53
  in Levine's conservation model, 94, 96-97
  in Neuman's systems model, 116-117, 121-122
Assessment questions in Neuman's systems model, 122-123
Authority in King's systems framework, 74

B

Becoming, human, theory of, 38
Behavioral assessment
  in Johnson's behavioral system model, 54, 56-57, 59-61
  in Roy's adaptation model, 179, 180, 182, 184, 185-186, 188-189, 191, 192, 194, 196
Behavioral system, theory of person as, 35
Behavioral system model, Johnson's; *see* Johnson's behavioral system model
Biological assessment in Johnson's behavioral system model, 62
Body image in King's systems framework, 73
Broad-range theories, 32-33

C

Case studies
  using Johnson's behavioral system model, 56-68
  using King's systems framework, 78-87
  using Levine's conservation model, 95-104
  using Neuman's systems model, 116-126
  using Orem's self-care deficit theory, 136-148
  using Rogers' science of unitary human beings, 164-172
  using Roy's adaptation model, 181-198
Change
  accelerating, theory of, 38
  knowing participation in, theory of power as, 159
  rhythmical correlates of, theory of, 38
Choice in Johnson's behavioral system model, 51
Client stability, optimal, theory of, 37
Client system in Neuman's systems model, 111, 112
Commonplaces of discipline in Levine's conservation model, 91
Communication in King's systems framework, 73
Conceptual environment in Levine's conservation model, 92
Conceptual models of nursing, nursing theories, and nursing practice, 33, 211-221
Conceptualization, 1-45
  critical thinking structures and, 31-45
  models and theories in nursing practice and, 15-30
  nursing knowledge and, 3-13
Confusion, perspective transformation and, 215
Consciousness, expanding, health as, theory of, 38
Conservation
  in Levine's conservation model, 90
  theory of, 36
Conservation model, Levine's; see Levine's conservation model
Control operations in Orem's self-care deficit theory, 135, 136, 142, 148
Coping in King's systems framework, 73
Correlates, rhythmical, of change, theory of, 38

Critical thinking, 40
  Johnson's behavioral system model and, 52-56
  in King's systems framework, 75-78
  in Levine's conservation model, 94-96
  models and theories and, 31-45
  in Neuman's systems model, 114-121
  in Orem's self-care deficit theory, 132-136
  relationship of, with nursing and trans-actions processes, 77
  in Rogers' science of unitary human beings, 159-165
  in Roy's adaptation model, 178-182
Cultural/social assessment in Johnson's behavioral system model, 61-62
Curriculum era of nursing knowledge, 4-5

D

DBSM; see Derdiarian Behavioral System model
Decision making in King's systems framework, 74, 75
Departmental power, theory of, 35
Dependency assessment in Johnson's behavioral system model, 60
Dependent-care deficit, theory of, 38
Derdiarian Behavioral System model (DBSM), 50
Development
  growth and, in King's systems framework, 73
  proximal, zone of, 65
Developmental assessment
  in Johnson's behavioral system model, 62
  in Neuman's systems model, 112, 117, 123
Diagnosis, nursing; see Nursing diagnosis
Diagnostic analysis in Johnson's behavioral system model, 54-55, 63-64
Diagnostic operations in Orem's self-care deficit theory, 134-135, 137-142, 143, 144-145, 146-147
Discipline, commonplaces of, in Levine's conservation model, 91
Discrepancy in Johnson's behavioral system model, 52
Dissonance
  perceived, theory of, 38, 157-159
  perspective transformation and, 214-215

Distress, spiritual, in Roy's adaptation model, 195-196

Documentation of nursing practice, 217-218

Dominance in Johnson's behavioral system model, 52

Dwelling with uncertainty, perspective transformation and, 215

E

Ecological assessment in Johnson's behavioral system model, 62

Eliminative assessment in Johnson's behavioral system model, 60-61

Energy conservation, 36
  in Levine's conservation model, 92, 96-97, 99, 102-103

Energy field in Rogers' science of unitary human beings, 38, 155

Environment
  assessment of, in Johnson's behavioral system model, 54, 57-58, 61-63
  in Levine's conservation model, 91
  in Rogers' science of unitary human beings, 156

Environmental field patterning in Rogers' science of unitary human beings, 160, 163

Evaluation
  in Johnson's behavioral system model, 55, 58-59, 68
  in Levine's conservation model, 95
  in Rogers' science of unitary human beings, 160, 163-164, 167-168
  in Roy's adaptation model, 180, 181, 183, 185, 188, 190, 192, 193-194, 196, 198

Expanding consciousness, health as, theory of, 38

Expansion, 201-221
  conceptual models of nursing and, 211-221
  further development of theory-based nursing practice and, 203-210

External environment in Levine's conservation model, 92

Extrapersonal stressor in Neuman's systems model, 112

F

Familial assessment in Johnson's behavioral system model, 61

Fibromyalgia (FM), 100-104

Field motion, human, theory of, 38

Flexible line of defense (FLD) in Neuman's systems model, 111-112

FM; see Fibromyalgia

Framework, 33, 39
  King's systems; see King's systems framework

Functional requirements of subsystems in Johnson's behavioral system model, 52

Fundamentals, nursing knowledge and, 5

G

General theory of nursing, 38

Goal attainment
  in King's systems framework, 72
  theory of, 35

Goal setting in Roy's adaptation model, 180, 181, 182-183, 185, 186-187, 189, 192, 193, 194, 197

Goals
  in Johnson's behavioral system model, 53-55
  for theoretical guidance in Orem's self-care deficit theory, 136-137

Graduate education era of nursing knowledge, 6-8

Grand theories, 32-33

Grief in Roy's adaptation model, 195

Growth and development in King's systems framework, 73

H

Health
  as expanding consciousness, theory of, 38
  in King's systems framework, 71
  in Levine's conservation model, 91
  social support and, theory of, 35

Helicy, in Rogers' science of unitary human beings, 38

HIV; see Human immunodeficiency virus

Homeless women, case study of, with Neuman's systems model, 120-126

Homeodynamic principles, in Rogers' science of unitary human beings, 38, 156-157

Human becoming, theory of, 38

Human field motion, theory of, 38

Human field patterning in Rogers' science of unitary human beings, 160, 162-163

Human immunodeficiency virus (HIV), 190-198

Hypotheses in Levine's conservation model, 95, 98, 102

I

Illness in Levine's conservation model, 92

Imperatives, sustenal; see Sustenal imperatives

Implementation in Roy's adaptation model, 183, 185, 187-188, 189-190, 192, 193, 194-196, 197

Incompatibility in Johnson's behavioral system model, 52

Ingestive assessment in Johnson's behavioral system model, 60

Instinctual knowledge in Rogers' science of unitary human beings, 161

Insufficiency in Johnson's behavioral system model, 52

Integrality in Rogers' science of unitary human beings, 38

Integrity, structural, conservation of, 36

Intention, therapeutic, theory of, 36

Interaction in King's systems framework, 73

Interdependence adaptive mode in Roy's adaptation model, 180, 184-185, 192-194

Interdependence mode, theory of, 39

International Orem Society for Scholarship and Nursing Science (IOS), 131

Interpersonal relationships in King's systems framework and theory, 71

Interpersonal stressor in Neuman's systems model, 112

Interpersonal system in King's systems framework and theory, 35, 72, 73

Interpretation in King's systems framework, 77

Intervention
  in Johnson's behavioral system model, 55, 64-67
  prevention as, theory of, 37
  in Roy's adaptation model, 180, 181

Intrapersonal stressor in Neuman's systems model, 112

Intuitive knowledge in Rogers' science of unitary human beings, 161

IOS; see International Orem Society for Scholarship and Nursing Science

J

JBSM; see Johnson's behavioral system model

Johnson, Dorothy E., 16, 17, 18, 34-35, 49-70, 176, 204, 205, 206, 207

Johnson's behavioral system model (JBSM), 16, 17, 18, 34-35, 49-70
  achievement assessment in, 59
  affiliative assessment in, 60
  aggressive/protective assessment in, 60
  behavioral assessment in, 54, 56-57, 59-61
  biological assessment in, 62
  case studies using, 56-68
  choice in, 51
  critical thinking in nursing practice with, 52-56
  cultural/social assessment in, 61-62
  dependency assessment in, 60
  developmental assessment in, 62
  diagnostic analysis in, 54-55, 63-64
  discrepancy in, 52
  dominance in, 52
  ecological assessment in, 62
  eliminative assessment in, 60-61
  environmental assessment in, 54, 57-58, 61-63
  evaluation in, 55, 58-59, 68
  familial assessment in, 61
  functional requirements of, 52
  further development of, 204, 205, 206, 207
  history and background of, 49-51
  incompatibility in, 52
  ingestive assessment in, 60
  insufficiency in, 52
  overview of, 51-52
  pathological assessment in, 62
  perseverative set in, 51
  planning and intervention in, 55, 64-67
  preparatory set in, 51
  protective/aggressive assessment in, 60
  psychological assessment in, 62-63
  restorative assessment in, 61
  set in, 51
  sexual assessment in, 61
  social/cultural assessment in, 61-62
  sustenal imperatives in, 52

Judgments in Levine's conservation model, 94, 97-98, 102

K

King, Imogene, 16, 17, 18, 35, 71-88, 205, 206-207

King's systems framework, 16, 17, 18, 35, 71-88
  authority in, 74
  body image in, 73
  case studies using, 78-87
  communication in, 73
  coping in, 73
  critical thinking in, 75-78
  decision making in, 74, 75
  further development of, 205, 206-207
  growth and development in, 73
  history and background of, 71-72
  interaction in, 73
  interpersonal systems in, 73
  learning in, 73
  organization in, 74
  overview of, 72-74
  perception in, 71, 72
  personal space in, 73, 84
  personal systems in, 72-73
  power in, 74
  relationships, interpersonal, in, 71
  role in, 73, 85
  self in, 73, 79, 83-84
  social systems in, 74, 75
  status in, 74
  stress in, 73
  stressors in, 73
  time in, 73, 84
  transaction in, 73

Knowing participation in change, theory of power as, 159

Knowledge, nursing; *see* Nursing knowledge

Kuhn's philosophy of science, 8

L

Learning in King's systems framework, 73

Levine, M.E., 16, 17, 18, 36, 89-107, 205, 206, 207

Levine's conservation model, 16, 17, 18, 36, 89-107
  assessment in, 94, 96-97
  case studies using, 95-104
  commonplaces of discipline in, 91
  conceptual environment in, 92
  critical thinking in, 94-96

Levine's conservation model—cont'd
  energy conservation in, 96-97, 99, 102-103
  evaluation in, 95
  external environment in, 92
  further development of, 205, 206, 207
  history and background of, 89-90
  hypotheses in, 95, 98, 102
  judgments in, 94, 97-98, 102
  nursing interventions in, 95, 98-99, 102-104
  operational environment in, 92
  organismic responses in, 99-100, 104
  overview of, 90-93
  perceptual environment in, 92
  personal integrity in, 97, 99, 104
  social integrity in, 97, 99, 104
  structural integrity in, 97, 99, 103-104
  theories for practice of, 93-94
  trophicognosis in, 94, 97-98, 102

Life-protecting buffer in Neuman's systems model, 112

Lines of resistance (LOR) in Neuman's systems model, 112

M

Meditation in Rogers' science of unitary human beings, 171

Metaparadigm, 33

Methodology for study of nursing process, 73

Middle-range theories, 32-33

Model, 39
  Johnson's behavioral system; *see* Johnson's behavioral system model
  Levine's conservation; *see* Levine's conservation model
  Neuman's systems; *see* Neuman's systems model
  Roy's adaptation; *see* Roy's adaptation model
  and theories
    critical thinking structures and, 31-45
    Johnson's behavioral system model, 34-35
    King's systems framework, 35
    Levine's conservation model, 36
    Neuman's systems model, 36-37
    in nursing practice, 15-30

Model—cont'd
  and theories—cont'd
    Orem's conceptual model, 37-38
    relationship of, 32-39
    Rogers' science of unitary human beings, 38
    Roy's adaptation model, 39
    selection of, 41-42
Mutual patterning in Rogers' science of unitary human beings, 160, 161-163, 166-167, 170-172

N

Neuman, B., 16, 17, 18, 36-37, 109-127, 205, 206, 207, 208
Neuman's systems model, 16, 17, 18, 36-37, 109-127
  assessment in, 116-117, 121-122
  assessment questions in, 122-123
  case studies using, 116-126
  client system in, 111, 112
  critical thinking in, 114-116
  developmental assessment in, 117, 122, 123
  extrapersonal stressor in, 112
  further development of, 205, 206, 207, 208
  history and background of, 109-110
  life-protecting buffer in, 112
  lines of resistance (LOR) in, 112
  organization of data in, 117-118
  overview of, 110-114
  physiological assessment in, 116, 121, 123
  prevention in, 113
  problem list in, 118-119, 123
  psychological assessment in, 116, 121, 123
  reflection on data in, 119-120, 123-125
  sociocultural assessment in, 116, 121-122, 123
  spiritual assessment in, 117, 122, 123
  synthesis and analysis of data in, 120, 125, 126
  throughput in, 110
  wholism in, 109
Neuropsychiatric Institute and Hospital Classification System, UCLA, 49-50
Normal line of defense (NLD) in Neuman's systems model, 111-112

Nurse Scientist Training Program, 6-7
Nursing
  conceptual models of, 211-221
  general theory of, 38
  in Levine's conservation model, 91
Nursing arts laboratory, 5
Nursing diagnosis
  in Johnson's behavioral system model, 53
  in Roy's adaptation model, 179, 180, 182, 184, 186, 189, 191-192, 193, 194, 196-197
Nursing interventions in Levine's conservation model, 95, 98-99, 102-104
Nursing knowledge
  curriculum era of, 4-5
  eras of, 4-10
  graduate education era of, 6-8
  nature of, needed for nursing practice, 3-13
  perspective transformation and, 214-217
  philosophic value of, 212-213
  research era of, 5-6
  scientific value of, 217-219
  theory era of, 8-10
Nursing knowledge–based nursing practice, implementation of, 213-217
Nursing practice
  centrality of, 10-11
  conceptual models of, 211-221
  documentation of, 217-218
  nature of knowledge needed for, 3-13
  nursing knowledge–based, implementation of, 213-217
  satisfaction with, 218-219
  scope and substance of, 218
  theories and models in, 15-30
  theory-based, areas for further development of, 203-210
Nursing process
  methodology for study of, 73
  relationship of, with critical thinking and transactions processes, 77
Nursing system
  in Orem's self-care deficit theory, 37, 38
  theory of, 38
Nursing theories, conceptual models of, 211-221

O

Openness in Rogers' science of unitary human beings, 38, 155

Operational environment in Levine's conservation model, 92

Optimal client stability, theory of, 37

Orem, D.E., 16, 17, 18, 37-38, 129-152, 205, 206, 207, 208

Orem's self-care deficit theory, 16, 17, 18, 37-38, 129-152

  case studies in, 136-148

  control operations in, 135, 136, 142, 148

  critical thinking in, 132-136

  diagnostic operations in, 134-135, 137-142, 143, 144-145, 146-147

  further development of, 205, 206, 207, 208

  goal for theoretical guidance in, 136-137

  history and background of, 129-131

  overview of, 131-132

  prescriptive operations in, 133, 134, 137-142, 143, 144-145, 146-147

  regulatory operations in, 133-136, 142, 148

Organismic responses in Levine's conservation model, 99-100, 104

Organization

  of data in Neuman's systems model, 117-118

  in King's systems framework, 74

Output in Neuman's systems model, 110

P

Pandimensionality in Rogers' science of unitary human beings, 38, 155-156

Paradigm, 33, 39

Paranormal phenomena, theory of, 38

Pathological assessment in Johnson's behavioral system model, 62

Pattern appraisal in Rogers' science of unitary human beings, 160-161, 165-166, 169-170

Patterning in Rogers' science of unitary human beings, 38, 155, 161-163

Perceived dissonance, theory of, 38, 157-159

Perception in King's systems framework, 71, 72

Perceptual environment in Levine's conservation model, 92

Perseverative set in Johnson's behavioral system model, 51

Person

  as adaptive system, theory of, 39

  in Levine's conservation model, 91

  theory of, as behavioral system, 35

Personal integrity

  conservation of, 36

  in Levine's conservation model, 92, 97, 99, 104

Personal space in King's systems framework, 73, 84

Personal system in King's systems framework, 35, 72-73

Perspective transformation, nursing knowledge and, 214-217

Phenomena, paranormal, theory of, 38

Philosophic value of nursing knowledge, 212-213

Physiological adaptive mode in Roy's adaptation model, 180, 182-183, 191-192

Physiological assessment in Neuman's systems model, 112, 116, 121, 123

Physiological mode, theory of, 39

Planning in Johnson's behavioral system model, 55, 64-67

Power

  departmental, theory of, 35

  in King's systems framework and theory, 74

  theory of, 38

    as knowing participation in change, 159

Preparatory set in Johnson's behavioral system model, 51

Prescriptive operations in Orem's self-care deficit theory, 133, 134, 137-142, 143, 144-145, 146-147

Prevention

  as intervention, theory of, 37

  in Neuman's systems model, 113

Primary prevention in Neuman's systems model, 113

Problem list in Neuman's systems model, 118-119, 123

Protective/aggressive assessment in Johnson's behavioral system model, 60

Proximal development, zone of, 65

Psychological assessment

  in Johnson's behavioral system model, 62-63

Psychological assessment—cont'd
  in Neuman's systems model, 112, 116, 121, 123

R

RAM; *see* Roy's adaptation model
Reconceptualization, perspective transformation and, 215-216
Redundancy, theory of, 36, 94
Reflection on data in Neuman's systems model, 119-120, 123-125
Regulatory operations in Orem's self-care deficit theory, 133-136, 142, 148
Relationships, interpersonal, in King's systems framework, 71
Research era of nursing knowledge, 5-6
Resolution, perspective transformation and, 215
Resonancy in Rogers' science of unitary human beings, 38
Restorative assessment in Johnson's behavioral system model, 61
Restorative subsystem, theory of, 35
Rhythmical correlates of change, theory of, 38
Rogers, Martha, 16, 17, 18, 38, 153-174, 205, 206, 207, 208-209
Rogers' science of unitary human beings, 16, 17, 18, 38, 153-174
  analysis and synthesis in, 164
  case studies using, 164-172
  critical thinking in, 159-165
  definition of unitary human being in, 156
  energy field in, 38, 155
  environment in, 156
  environmental field patterning in, 160, 163
  evaluation in, 160, 163-164, 167-168
  further development of, 205, 206, 207, 208-209
  helicy in, 38
  history and background of, 153-155
  homeodynamic principles in, 156-157
  human field patterning in, 160, 162-163
  instinctual knowledge in, 161
  integrality in, 38
  meditation in, 171
  mutual patterning in, 160, 161-163, 166-167, 170-172

Rogers' science of unitary human beings—cont'd
  openness in, 38, 155
  overview of, 155-157
  pandimensionality in, 155-156
  pattern appraisal in, 160-161, 165-166, 169-170
  patterning in, 38, 155, 161-163
  resonancy in, 38
  theories for practice in, 157-159
  theory of perceived dissonance in, 157-159
  theory of power as knowing participation in change in, 159
  touch, therapeutic, in, 167
Role function adaptive mode in Roy's adaptation model, 180, 188-191, 196-198
Role function mode, theory of, 39
Role in King's systems framework, 73, 85
Roy, Sr. Callista, 7, 16, 17, 18, 39, 175-200, 205, 206, 207, 209
Roy's adaptation model (RAM), 16, 17, 18, 39, 175-200
  behavioral assessment in, 179, 180, 182, 184, 185-186, 188-189, 191, 192, 194, 196
  case studies using, 181-198
  critical thinking in, 178-182
  evaluation in, 180, 181, 183, 185, 188, 190, 192, 193-194, 196, 198
  further development of, 205, 206, 207, 209
  goal setting in, 180, 181, 182-183, 185, 186-187, 189, 192, 193, 194, 197
  grief in, 195
  history and background of, 176
  implementation in, 183, 185, 187-188, 189-190, 192, 193, 194-196, 197
  interdependence adaptive mode in, 180, 184-185, 192-194
  intervention in, 180, 181
  nursing diagnosis in, 179, 180, 182, 184, 186, 189, 191-192, 193, 194, 196-197
  overview of, 176-178
  physiological adaptive mode in, 180, 182-183, 191-192
  role function adaptive mode in, 188-191, 196-198

Roy's adaptation model (RAM)—cont'd
  self-concept adaptive mode in, 180, 185-188, 194-196
  sexual dysfunction in, 196
  spiritual distress in, 195-196
  stimuli assessment in, 179, 180, 182, 184, 186, 189, 191, 192, 194, 196

S

Satisfaction with nursing practice, 218-219
Saturation, perspective transformation and, 215
SCDNT; *see* Self-care deficit nursing theory
Science of unitary human beings, Rogers'; *see* Rogers' science of unitary human beings
Scientific value of nursing knowledge, 217-219
Secondary prevention in Neuman's systems model, 113
Self in King's systems framework, 73, 79, 83-84
Self-care
  in Orem's self-care deficit theory, 37, 38
  theory of, 38
Self-care deficit in Orem's self-care deficit theory, 37, 38
Self-care deficit nursing theory (SCDNT), 38, 129-152
  Orem's; *see* Orem's self-care deficit theory
Self-concept adaptive mode in Roy's adaptation model, 180, 185-188, 194-196
Self-concept mode, theory of, 39
Set in Johnson's behavioral system model, 51
Sexual assessment in Johnson's behavioral system model, 61
Sexual dysfunction in Roy's adaptation model, 196
Skills laboratories, 5
Social integrity
  conservation of, 36
  in Levine's conservation model, 92, 97, 99, 104
Social support and health, theory of, 35
Social systems in King's systems framework, 35, 71, 72, 74, 75
Sociocultural assessment
  in Johnson's behavioral system model, 61-62

Sociocultural assessment—cont'd
  in Neuman's systems model, 112, 116, 121-122, 123
Spiritual assessment in Neuman's systems model, 112, 117, 123
Spiritual distress in Roy's adaptation model, 195-196
Stability
  optimal client theory of, 37
  perspective transformation and, 214
Status in King's systems framework, 74
Stimulus
  assessment of, in Roy's adaptation model, 179, 180, 182, 184, 186, 189, 191, 192, 194, 196
  in Roy's adaptation model, 175
Stress in King's systems framework, 73
Stressor
  extrapersonal, 112
  intrapersonal, 112
  in King's systems framework, 73
Structural integrity
  conservation of, 36
  in Levine's conservation model, 97, 99, 103-104
Subsystem
  in Johnson's behavioral system model, 51-52
  in Neuman's systems model, 110
Sustenal imperatives
  in Johnson's behavioral system model, 52
  theory of, 35
Synthesis
  and analysis of data
    in Neuman's systems model, 120, 125, 126
    in Rogers' science of unitary human beings, 164
  in King's systems framework, 77
  perspective transformation and, 215
Systems framework, King's; *see* King's systems framework
Systems model, Neuman's; *see* Neuman's systems model

T

Tertiary prevention in Neuman's systems model, 113
Theory, 33
  of accelerating change, 38

Theory—cont'd
    of aging, 38
    broad-range, 32-33
    of conservation, 36
    of departmental power, 35
    of dependent-care deficit, 38
    general, of nursing, 38
    of goal attainment, 35
    grand, 32-33
    of health as expanding consciousness, 38
    of human becoming, 38
    of human field motion, 38
    of interdependence mode, 39
    King's systems framework and; *see*
        King's systems framework
    middle-range, 32-33
    and models; *see* Model and theories
    of nursing systems, 38
    of optimal client stability, 37
    Orem's self-care deficit; *see* Orem's self-
        care deficit theory
    of paranormal phenomena, 38
    of perceived dissonance, 38, 157-159
    of person
        as adaptive system, 39
        as behavioral system, 35
    of physiological mode, 39
    of power, 38
        as knowing participation in change,
            159
    of prevention as intervention, 37
    of redundancy, 36, 94
    of restorative subsystem, 35
    of rhythmical correlates of change, 38
    of role function mode, 39
    of self-care, 38
    self-care deficit, 38
    of self-concept mode, 39
    of social support and health, 35
    of sustenal imperatives, 35
    of therapeutic intention, 36

Theory era of nursing knowledge, 8-10
Theory-based nursing practice, areas for
        further development of, 203-210
Therapeutic intention, theory of, 36
Therapeutic touch in Rogers' science of
        unitary human beings, 167
Thinking, critical; *see* Critical thinking
Throughput in Neuman's systems model,
        110
Time in King's systems framework, 73, 84
Touch, therapeutic, in Rogers' science of
        unitary human beings, 167
Transaction
    in King's systems framework, 73
    relationship of, with nursing and critical
        thinking processes, 77
Trophicognosis in Levine's conservation
        model, 94, 97-98, 102

U

UCLA Neuropsychiatric Institute and Hos-
        pital Classification System, 49-50
Uncertainty, dwelling with, perspective
        transformation and, 215
Unitary human beings, Rogers' science of,
        38, 153-174

V

Vygotsky's zone of proximal development,
        65

W

Wholeness in Levine's conservation model,
        90, 91
Wholism in Neuman's systems model, 109

Z

Zone of proximal development (ZPD), 65